ABC
ARTERIAL AND V

ABC OF
ARTERIAL AND VENOUS DISEASE

edited by

RICHARD DONNELLY

Professor of Vascular Medicine,
University of Nottingham and Southern Derbyshire Acute Hospitals NHS Trust, Derby, UK

and

NICK J M LONDON

Professor of Surgery, University of Leicester, UK

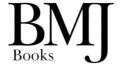

© BMJ Books 2000
BMJ Books is an imprint of the BMJ Publishing Group

First published in 2000
by BMJ Books, BMA House, Tavistock Square,
London WC1H 9JR

www.bmjbooks.com

British Library Cataloguing in Publication Data
A catalogue record for this book is available from the British Library

ISBN 0-7279-1561-4

Cover design by Marritt Associates, Harrow, Middlesex
Composition by Scribe Design, Gillingham, Kent
Printed and bound in Spain by GraphyCems

Contents

Contributors

D Adu
Consultant Physician, Queen Elizabeth Hospital, Birmingham

Philip MW Bath
Professor of Stroke Medicine, University of Nottingham, Nottingham

Jonathan D Beard
Consultant Vascular Surgeron, Sheffield Vascular Institute, Northern General Hospital, Sheffield

PRF Bell
Professor of Surgery, University of Leicester, Lericester

Andrew Bradbury
Professor of Surgery, University of Birmingham, Birmingham Heartlands Hospital, Birmingham

Ken Callum
Consultant Surgeon, Derbyshire Royal Infirmary, Derby

P Cockwell
Consultant Physician, Queen Elizabeth Hospital, Birmingham

Karl R Davis
Clinical Research Fellow, Southern Derbyshire Acute Hospitals NHS Trust, Derby

Richard Donnelly
Professor of Vascular Medicine, University of Nottingham and Southern Derbyshire Acute Hospitals NHS Trust, Derby

Alistair M Emslie-Smith
General Practitioner, Tayside Centre for General Practice, Dundee

Fiona Fennessy
Research Fellow, Beaumont Hospital, Dublin, Ireland

Iain D Gardner
Consultant Ophthalmologist, Derbyshire Royal Infirmary, Derby

W Peter Gorman
Consultant Physician, Southern Derbyshire Acute Hospitals NHS Trust, Derby

L Harper
Specialist Registrar, Queen Elizabeth Hospital, Birmingham

David Bouchier Hayes
Professor of Surgery, Beaumont Hospital, Dublin, Ireland

David Hinwood
Consultant Vascular Radiologist, Derbyshire Royal Infirmary, Derby

A Howic
Reader in Renal Pathology, University of Birmingham, Birmingham

Alan G Jardine
Senior Lecturer and Consultant Nephrologist, Department of Medicine and Therapeutics, Western Infirmary, Glasgow

Kennedy R Lees
Professor of Cerebrovascular Medicine, University Department of Medicine and Therapeutics, Western Infirmary, Glasgow

Nick JM London
Professor of Surgery, University of Leicester, Leicester

Kevin McLaughlin
Assistant Professor in Nephrology, University of Calgary, Canada

Peter S Mortimer
Consultant Skin Physician, St george's Hospital and Royal Marsden Hospital, London

Jon G Moss
Consultant Interventional Radiologist, Gartnavel General Hospital, Glasgow

Andrew D Morris
Senior Lecturer in Medicine and Diabetes, Ninewells Hospital and Medical School, Dundee

Roddy Nash
Consultant Surgeon, Derbyshire Royal Infirmary, Derby

A Ross Naylor
Senior Lecturer, Department of Surgery, Leicester Royal Infirmary, Leicester

COS Savage
Professor of Nephrology, University of Birmingham, Birmingham

Sean Tierney
Lecturer in Surgery, Beaumont Hospital, Dublin, Ireland

MM Thompson
Consultant Vascular and Endovascular Surgeon, Leicester Royal Infirmary, Leicester

Preface

The clinical manifestations of arterial and venous disease are often the result of various pathophysiological mechanisms, including atherosclerosis, thrombosis, inflammation, embolism and aneurysm formation. Despite the varied aetiology, modern developments in noninvasive imaging, particularly duplex scanning, have revolutionised the clinical approach to identifying structural and functional abnormalities in peripheral arteries and veins.

The authorship of these chapters reflects a more integrated approach to clinical management involving surgeons, physicians, radiologists and vascular laboratory technicians working closely to achieve optimum outcomes. For example, the approach to carotid disease and renal artery stenosis demonstrates the importance of multidisciplinary input to clinical decision making.

The subject areas covered in this series lend themselves to illustration, and the photographs, radiological images and tables will be particularly helpful to the non-specialist reader. Wherever possible, we have tried to ensure that clinical practice recommendations in this book are evidence based, but clinical trials in patients with arterial and venous disease have been relatively limited and there are still gaps in our knowledge. Nevertheless, this book provides an up to date text covering best practice in a rapidly changing and diverse group of common clinical disorders.

Richard Donnelly
University of Nottingham
Nick J M London
University of Leicester

1 Non-invasive methods of arterial and venous assessment

Richard Donnelly, David Hinwood, Nick J M London

Although diagnostic and therapeutic decisions in patients with vascular disease are guided primarily by the history and physical examination, the use of non-invasive investigations has increased significantly in recent years, mainly as a result of technological advances in ultrasonography. This article describes the main investigative techniques.

Principles of vascular ultrasonography

In the simplest form of ultrasonography, ultrasound is transmitted as a continuous beam from a probe that contains two piezoelectric crystals. The transmitting crystal produces ultrasound at a fixed frequency (set by the operator according to the depth of the vessel being examined), and the receiving crystal vibrates in response to reflected waves and produces an output voltage. Conventional B mode (brightness mode) ultrasonography records the ultrasound waves reflected from tissue interfaces, and a two dimensional picture is built up according to the reflective properties of the tissues.

Doppler ultrasonography
Ultrasound signals reflected off stationary surfaces retain the same frequency with which they were transmitted, but the principle underlying Doppler ultrasonography is that the frequency of signals reflected from moving objects such as red blood cells shifts in proportion to the velocity of the target. The output from a continuous wave Doppler ultrasonograph is usually presented as an audible signal, so that a sound is heard whenever there is movement of blood in the vessel being examined.

Pulsed ultrasonography
Continuous wave ultrasonography provides little scope for restricting the area of tissue that is being examined because any sound waves that are intercepted by the receiving crystal will produce an output signal. The solution is to use pulsed ultrasonography. The investigator can focus on a specific tissue plane by transmitting a pulse of ultrasound and closing the receiver except when signals from a predetermined depth are returning. This allows, for example, the centre of an artery and the areas close to the vessel wall to be examined in turn.

Duplex scanners
An important advance in vascular ultrasonography has been the development of spectral analysis, which delineates the complete spectrum of frequencies (that is, blood flow velocities) found in the arterial waveform during a single cardiac cycle. The normal ("triphasic") Doppler velocity waveform is made up of three components which correspond to different phases of arterial flow: rapid antegrade flow reaching a peak during systole, transient reversal of flow during early diastole, and slow antegrade flow during late diastole.

Doppler examination of an artery distal to a stenosis will show characteristic changes in the velocity profile: the rate of rise is delayed, the amplitude decreased, and the transient flow reversal in early diastole is lost. In severe disease, the Doppler

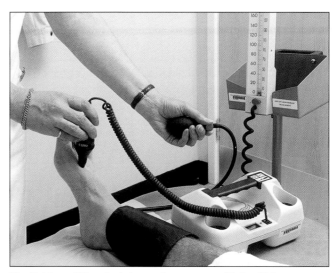

Handheld pencil Doppler being used to measure ankle brachial pressure index

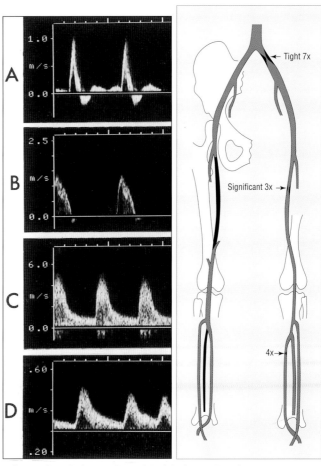

Left: Doppler velocity waveforms: (*a*) triphasic waveform in normal artery; (*b*) biphasic waveform, with increased velocity, through a mild stenosis; (*c*) monophasic waveform, with greatly increased velocity, through tight stenosis; and (*d*) dampened monophasic waveform, with reduced velocity, recorded distal to tight stenosis. Right: Anatomical chart used to record position of stenoses, showing three stenoses with velocity increases of 7×, 4×, and 3× compared with adjacent unaffected arteries

waveform flattens; in critical limb ischaemia it may be undetectable.

Examination of an arterial stenosis shows an increase in blood velocity through the area of narrowing. The site(s) of any stenotic lesions can be identified by serial placement of the Doppler probe along the extremities. The criteria used to define a stenosis vary between laboratories, but a twofold increase in peak systolic velocity compared with the velocity in an adjacent segment of the artery usually signifies a stenosis of 50% or more.

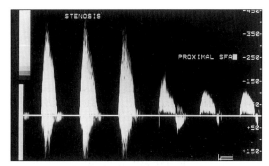

Relation between increased blood velocity and degree of stenosis

Diameter of stenosis (%)	Peak sytolic velocity* (m/s)	Peak diastolic velocity* (m/s)	Internal: common carotid artery velocity ratio†
0-39	< 1.1	< 0.45	< 1.8
4-59	1.1-1.49	< 0.45	< 1.8
60-79	1.5-2.49	0.45-1.4	1.8-3.7
80-99	2.5-6.1	> 1.4	> 3.7
> 99 (critical)	Extremely low	NA	NA

*Measured in lower part of internal carotid artery
†Ratio of peak systolic velocity in internal carotid artery stenosis relative to proximal measurement in common carotid artery

By combining the pulsed Doppler system with real time B mode ultrasound imaging of vessels, it is possible to examine Doppler flow patterns in a precisely defined area within the vessel lumen. This combination of real time B mode sound imaging with pulsed Doppler ultrasonography is called duplex scanning. The addition of colour frequency mapping (so called colour duplex or triplex scanners) makes the identification of arterial stenoses even easier and reduces the scanning time.

Investigations of arterial disease

Ankle brachial pressure index
Under normal conditions, systolic blood pressure in the legs is equal to or slightly greater than the systolic pressure in the upper limbs. In the presence of an arterial stenosis, a reduction in pressure occurs distal to the lesion. The ankle brachial pressure index, which is calculated from the ratio of ankle to brachial systolic pressure, is a sensitive marker of arterial insufficiency.

The highest pressure measured in any ankle artery is used as the numerator in the calculation of the index; a value ≥ 1.0 is normal and a value < 0.9 is abnormal. Patients with claudication tend to have ankle brachial pressure indexes in the range 0.5-0.9, whereas those with critical ischaemia usually have an index of < 0.5. The index also has prognostic significance because of the association with arterial disease elsewhere, especially coronary heart disease.

Diabetic limbs
Systolic blood pressure in the lower limbs cannot be measured reliably when the vessels are calcified and incompressible—for example, in patients with diabetes—as this can result in falsely high ankle pressures. An alternative approach is to use either the pole test or measurement of toe pressures. Normal toe systolic pressure ranges from 90-100 mm Hg and is 80-90% of brachial systolic pressure. A toe systolic pressure < 30 mm Hg indicates critical ischaemia.

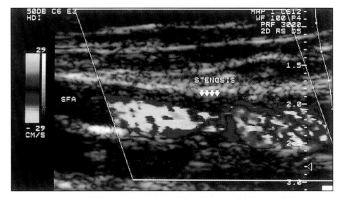

Spectral analysis of blood velocity in a stenosis, and unaffected area of proximal superficial femoral artery. The velocity increases from 150 to 300 m/s across the stenosis

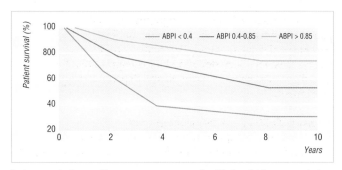

Colour duplex scanning of blood flow through stenosis of superficial femoral artery. Colour assignment (red or blue) depends on direction of blood flow and colour saturation reflects velocity of blood flow. Less saturation indicates regions of higher blood flow and deeper colours indicate slower flow; the absence of flow is coded as black

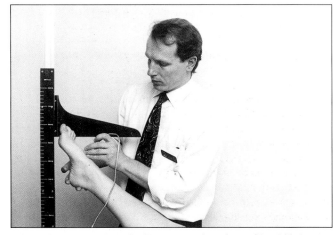

Patient survival according to measurements of ankle brachial pressure index (adapted from McKenna et al, *Atherosclerosis* 1991;87:119-28)

Pole test for measurement of ankle pressures in patients with calcified vessels: the Doppler probe is placed over a patent pedal artery and the foot raised against a pole that is calibrated in mm Hg. The point at which the pedal signal disappears is taken as the ankle pressure

Walk test

Exercise testing will assess the functional limitations of arterial stenoses and differentiate occlusive arterial disease from other causes of exercise induced lower limb symptoms—for example, neurogenic claudication secondary to spinal stenosis. A limited inflow of blood in a limb with occlusive arterial disease results in a fall in ankle systolic blood pressure during exercise induced peripheral vasodilatation.

The walk test is performed by exercising the patient for 5 minutes, ideally on a treadmill, but walking the patient in the surgery or marking time on the spot are adequate. The ankle brachial pressure index is measured before and after exercise. A pressure drop of 20% or more indicates significant arterial disease. If there is no drop in ankle systolic pressure after a 5 minute brisk walk, the patient does not have occlusive arterial disease proximal to the ankle in that limb.

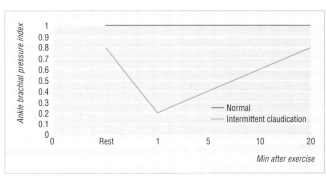

Fall in ankle brachial pressure index with exercise in patient with intermittent claudication and normal subject (adapted from Creager, *Vasc Med* 1997;2:231-7)

Duplex scanning

Duplex ultrasonography has a sensitivity of 80% and a specificity of 90-100% for detecting femoral and popliteal disease compared with angiography, but it is less reliable for assessing the severity of stenoses in the tibial and peroneal arteries. Duplex scanning is especially useful for assessing the carotid arteries and for surveillance of infrainguinal bypass grafts where sites of stenosis can be identified before complete graft occlusion occurs and before there is a fall in ankle brachial pressure index. The normal velocity within a graft conduit is 50-120 cm/s. As with native arteries, a twofold increase in peak systolic velocity indicates a stenosis of 50% or more. A peak velocity <45 cm/s occurs in grafts at high risk of failure.

Identification of distal vessels for arterial bypass grafting

In critically ischaemic limbs, where occlusive disease tends to be present at multiple levels, arteriography often fails to show patent calf or pedal vessels as potential outflows for femorodistal bypass grafting. Alternative non-invasive approaches have been developed for preoperative assessment, including pulse generated run off and dependent Doppler assessment.

Transcranial Doppler ultrasonography

Lower frequency Doppler probes (1-2 MHz) can be used to obtain information about blood flow in arteries comprising the circle of Willis and its principal branches. Mean flow velocities >80 cm/s in the middle cerebral artery, or >70 cm/s in the posterior and basilar arteries, indicate a serious stenosis. Transcranial Doppler scanning has several applications but is especially useful for intraoperative and postoperative monitoring of patients having carotid endarterectomy.

Helical or spiral computed tomography

Spiral computed tomography is a new, minimally invasive technique for vascular imaging that is made possible by combining two recent advances: slip ring computed tomography (which allows the *x* ray tube detector apparatus to rotate continuously) and computerised three dimensional reconstruction. A helical scan can cover the entire region of interest (for example, the abdominal aorta from the diaphragm to the iliac bifurcation) in one 30-40 second exposure, usually in a single breath hold. This minimises motion artefact and allows all the scan data to be collected during the first pass of an intravenous bolus of contrast through the arterial tree—that is during the time of maximal arterial opacification. A large number of finely spaced slices from one scan can then be reconstructed to produce high quality two or three dimensional images of the contrast enhanced vessels.

Uses of colour duplex scanning

Arterial	Venous
• Identify obstructive atherosclerotic disease: Carotid Renal	• Diagnosis of deep vein thrombosis above the knee
• Surveillance of infrainguinal bypass grafts	• Assessing competence of valves in deep veins
• Surveillance of lower limb arteries after angioplasty	• Superficial venous reflux: Assessing patient with recurrent varicose veins Identify and locate reflux at saphenopopliteal junction
	• Preoperative mapping of saphenous vein

Clinical use of transcranial Doppler scanning in adults

- Intraoperative monitoring during carotid endarterctomy:
  Shunt function
  Cerebral perfusion
- Postoperative montoring after carotid endarterectomy:
  Detection of emboli
  Formation of carotid thrombus
- Detection of intracranial vasospasm after subarachnoid haemorrhage
- Detection of middle cerebral artery disease
- Evaluation of collateral circulation in patients with carotid disease
- Evaluation of arteriovenous malformations of the brain

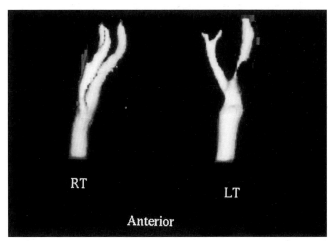

Spiral computed tomogram of both carotid systems showing a tight stenosis in the proximal segment of left internal carotid artery

Magnetic resonance angiography

Magnetic resonance angiography has developed rapidly over the past five years. It has the advantage of imaging a moving column of blood and does not require ionising radiation or iodinated contrast, but the technique has obvious drawbacks in terms of cost efficiency and accessibility to scanners. A variety of imaging sequences are used depending on the vessels being studied and the field strength of the machine. The most commonly used techniques include time of flight, two and three dimensional angiography and phase contrast.

Use of a magnetic resonance imaging scanner with a high field strength (which allows rapid acquisition of data) and a carefully timed bolus of gadolinium contrast enables high quality angiographic images to be obtained in a single breath hold. Magnetic resonance angiography is well established for examining the cerebral vessels and the carotid arteries, and its role in other territories is being extended.

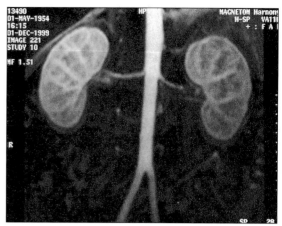

Magnetic resonance angiogram using an intravenous bolus of gadolinium contrast showing normal renal arteries

Investigations of venous disease

Venous thrombosis

Colour Duplex scanning is both sensitive and specific (90-100% in most series) for detecting proximal deep vein thrombosis. Deep veins and arteries lie together in the leg, and the normal vein appears as an echo-free channel and is usually larger than the accompanying artery.

Venous ultrasonography is a very accurate method of identifying deep vein thrombi from the level of the common femoral vein at the groin crease to the popliteal vein but is less reliable for diagnosing calf vein thrombosis.

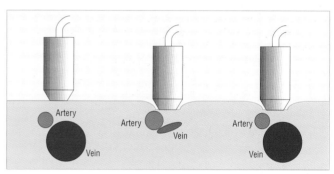

Ultrasound detection of deep vein thrombosis. The probe is held lightly on the skin and advanced along the course of the vein (left). Pressure is applied every few centimetres by compressing the transducer head against the skin. The vein collapses during compression if no thrombus is present (middle) but not if a deep vein thrombus is present (right)

Criteria for diagnosis of deep vein thrombosis

- Failure of vein to collapse on direct compression
- Visualisation of thrombus within lumen
- Absent or abnormal venous pulsation on Doppler scanning

Venous reflux

Colour duplex scanning has revolutionised the investigation of the lower limb venous system because it allows instant visualisation of blood flow and its direction. Thus, reflux at the saphenofemoral junction, saphenopopliteal junction, and within the deep venous system, including the popliteal vein beneath the knee and the gastrocnemius veins, can be detected without invasive techniques. Although venous reflux can be assessed with a pencil Doppler, this technique misses 12% of saphenofemoral and 20% of saphenopopliteal junction reflux compared with colour duplex scanning.

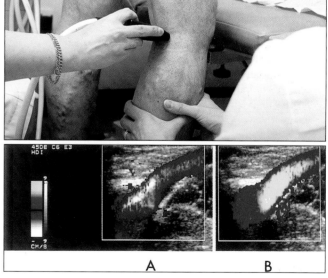

Colour duplex scanning of saphenopopliteal junction. The calf muscles are manually compressed producing upward flow in the vein (top), which appears as a blue colour for flow towards the heart (panel A). Sudden release of the distal compression causes reflux, seen as a red colour indicating flow away from the heart (panel B)

We thank Jean Clarke for expert secretarial assistance; Frances Ryan and Tim Hartshorne (vascular technicians) and colleagues in the vascular laboratories at Derbyshire Royal Infirmary and Leicester Royal Infirmary; Ken Callum and Roddy Nash (vascular surgeons) for helpful input to the manuscript and illustrations; and Jane Wain and staff of the audiovisual department at Derbyshire Royal Infirmary.

2 Acute limb ischaemia

Ken Callum, Andrew Bradbury

Limb ischaemia is classified on the basis of onset and severity. Complete acute ischaemia will lead to extensive tissue necrosis within six hours unless the limb is surgically revascularised. Incomplete acute ischaemia can usually be treated medically in the first instance. Patients with irreversible ischaemia require urgent amputation unless it is too extensive or the patient too ill to survive.

Clinical features

Apart from paralysis (inability to wiggle toes or fingers) and anaesthesia (loss of light touch over the dorsum of the foot or hand), the symptoms and signs of acute ischaemia are non-specific or inconsistently related to its completeness. Pain on squeezing the calf indicates muscle infarction and impending irreversible ischaemia.

Acute arterial occlusion is associated with intense spasm in the distal arterial tree, and initially the limb will appear "marble" white. Over the next few hours, the spasm relaxes and the skin fills with deoxygenated blood leading to mottling that is light blue or purple, has a fine reticular pattern, and blanches on pressure. At this stage the limb is still salvageable. However, as ischaemia progresses, stagnant blood coagulates leading to mottling that is darker in colour, coarser in pattern, and does not blanch. Finally, large patches of fixed staining progress to blistering and liquefaction. Attempts to revascularise such a limb are futile and will lead to life threatening reperfusion injury. In cases of real doubt the muscle can be examined at surgery through a small fasciotomy incision. It is usually obvious when the muscle is dead.

Aetiology

Acute limb ischaemia is most commonly caused by acute thrombotic occlusion of a pre-existing stenotic arterial segment (60% of cases) or by embolus (30%). Distinguishing these two conditions is important because treatment and prognosis are different. Other causes are trauma, iatrogenic injury, popliteal aneurysm, and aortic dissection.

More than 80% of peripheral emboli arise from the left atrial appendage in association with atrial fibrillation. They may also arise from the left ventricle, heart valves, prosthetic bypass grafts, aneurysmal disease, paradoxical embolism, and atrial myxoma (rare). In 15% of cases the source of embolus is obscure. Thrombosis in situ may arise from acute plaque rupture, hypovolaemia, or pump failure (see below).

Management

General measures

When a patient is suspected to have an acutely ischaemic limb the case must be discussed immediately with a vascular surgeon. A few hours can make the difference between death or amputation and complete recovery of limb function. If there are no contraindications (acute aortic dissection or multiple trauma, particularly serious head injury) give an intravenous bolus of heparin to limit propagation of thrombus and protect the collateral circulation.

Classification of limb ischaemia

Terminology	Definition or comment
Onset:	
Acute	Ischaemia < 14 days
Acute on chronic	Worsening symptoms and signs (< 14 days)
Chronic	Ischaemia stable for > 14 days
Severity (acute, acute on chronic):	
Incomplete	Limb not threatened
Complete	Limb threatened
Irreversible	Limb non-viable

Symptoms and signs of acute limb ischaemia

Symptoms or signs	Comment
Pain	Occasionally absent in complete ischaemia
Pallor	Also present in chronic ischaemia
Pulseless	Also present in chronic ischaemia
Perishing cold	Unreliable as ischaemic limb takes on ambient temperature
Paraesthesia*	Leading to anaesthesia (unable to feel touch on foot or hand)
Paralysis*	Unable to wiggle toes or fingers

*Anaesthesia and paralysis are the key to diagnosing complete ischaemia that requires emergency surgical treatment

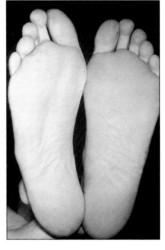

Marble white foot (left of picture) in patient with acute ischaemia

Differentiation of embolus and acute arterial thrombosis (thrombosis in situ)

Clinical features	Embolus	Thrombosis
Severity	Complete (no collaterals)	Incomplete (collaterals)
Onset	Seconds or minutes	Hours or days
Limb affected	Leg 3:1 arm	Leg 10:1 arm
Multiple sites	Up to 15%	Rare
Embolic source	Present (usually atrial fibrillation)	Absent
Previous claudication	Absent	Present
Palpation of artery	Soft, tender	Hard, calcified
Bruits	Absent	Present
Contralateral leg pulses	Present	Absent
Diagnosis	Clinical	Angiography
Treatment	Embolectomy, warfarin	Medical, bypass, thrombolysis

Is angiography required?

If ischaemia is complete, the patient must be taken directly to the operating theatre because angiography will introduce delay, thrombolysis is not an option, and lack of collateral flow will prevent visualisation of the distal vasculature. If ischaemia is incomplete the patient should have preoperative angiography since simple embolectomy or thrombectomy is unlikely to be successful, thrombolysis may be an option, and the surgeon requires a "road map" for distal bypass.

Acute embolus

Embolic occlusion of the brachial artery is not usually limb threatening, and in elderly people non-operative treatment is reasonable. Younger patients should have embolectomy to prevent subsequent claudication, especially if the dominant arm is affected.

A leg affected by embolus is nearly always threatened and requires immediate surgical revascularisation. Emboli usually lodge at the common femoral bifurcation or, less commonly, the popliteal trifurcation. Femoral embolus is associated with profound ischaemia to the level of the upper thigh because the deep femoral artery is also affected. A femoral pulse does not exclude the diagnosis. Embolectomy can be done under local, regional, or general anaesthetic.

The adequacy of embolectomy should be confirmed by angiography while the patient is on the operating table. On-table thrombolysis should be considered if mechanical clearance has been unsuccessful. If the embolus has occurred in an area of longstanding atherosclerotic disease, surgical bypass may be necessary.

Postoperatively the patient should continue to receive heparin to prevent formation of further emboli. Many surgeons postpone heparin for six hours after surgery to reduce the risk of a haematoma forming. Warfarin reduces the risk of recurrent embolism, and unless contraindicated, should be prescribed to all patients long term. Patients should not be given warfarin without first being on heparin for 48 hours since warfarin can produce a transient procoagulant state due to inhibition of the vitamin K dependent anticoagulant proteins C and S.

Opinions differ about how thorough you should be in establishing the source of emboli. Transthoracic echocardiography is poor at detecting a thrombus in patients with atrial fibrillation, and a negative result does not exclude the diagnosis. Transoesophageal echocardiography provides excellent views of the left atrium but is moderately invasive and not universally available. In patients with suspected paroxysmal tachyarrhythmias, 24 hour electrocardiographic monitoring should be considered. Even if no source of embolism is found, anticoagulation should continue long term.

Although immediate loss of a limb after correctly managed acute embolus is unusual, many series report a 10-20% in-hospital mortality from heart failure or recurrent embolism, particularly stroke.

Saddle embolus

Patients with acute embolic occlusion of the aortic bifurcation have no femoral pulses and appear marble white or mottled to the waist. They may also present with paraplegia due to ischaemia of the cauda equina, which can be irreversible. Immediate bilateral embolectomy restores lower limb perfusion, but many patients subsequently die from reperfusion injury.

Popliteal aneurysm

A popliteal aneurysm can initiate acute ischaemia by forming a thrombus or acting as a source of emboli. Thrombolysis is often the best treatment as simple embolectomy or thrombectomy

Factors predisposing to acute thrombosis	
Cause	**Comment**
Dehydration	Hot weather, diabetes, infection, gastroenteritis
Hypotension	Myocardial infarction, arrhythmia, heart failure, gastrointestinal haemorrhage, septic shock, multiple organ failure
Unusual posture or activity	Prolonged sitting, kneeling
Malignancy	Solid and haematological
Hyperviscosity	Polycythaemia, thrombocytosis
Thrombophilia	Protein C or S and antithrombin III deficiencies; activated protein C resistance; factor V Leiden; antiphospholipid syndrome

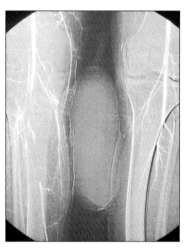

Embolus at popliteal trifurcation

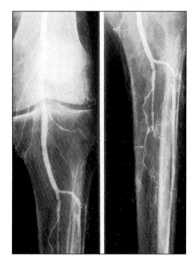

On-table angiograms showing incomplete clearance of embolus

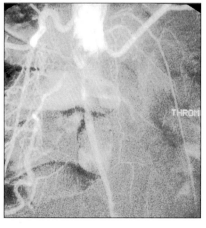

Aortic occlusion

usually leads to early rethrombosis and surgical bypass is often precluded by obliteration of the distal run-off. Once the circulation is restored, a bypass should be performed to exclude the aneurysm.

Atheroembolism
Cholesterol emboli are shed from a complex, often acutely ruptured, atherosclerotic plaque. Distal pulses are usually present. The patient characteristically presents with the blue toe (finger) syndrome, which may mimic Raynaud's phenomenon. If the blue toe syndrome is not recognised patients may deteriorate rapidly and require amputation.

Thrombosis in situ
Limbs affected by stable chronic ischaemia do not usually suddenly deteriorate without a reason—for example, silent myocardial infarction or underlying, hitherto asymptomatic, malignancy. Septicaemia, particularly pneumococcal and meningococcal, may be associated with widespread thrombosis.

Trauma
The commonest causes of non-iatrogenic injury are limb fractures and dislocations (supracondylar fractures of the humerus in children, tibial fractures in adults), blunt injuries occurring in road traffic accidents, and stab wounds. In the United Kingdom, acute traumatic limb ischaemia is often iatrogenic, being caused by arterial cannulation (coronary angioplasty, aortic balloon pump), vascular and orthopaedic procedures on the limb (especially if exsanguinating tourniquets are used), or pelvic surgery (cystectomy, anterior resection) in patients with subclinical aortoiliac disease in whom the ligated pelvic collaterals form the main blood supply to the legs. Postoperative assessment of lower limb ischaemia may be confused by the presence of epidural or spinal anaesthesia.

The presence of distal pulses does not exclude serious arterial injury. Pulse oximetry, Doppler signals, and measurement of the ankle brachial pressure index may be helpful, but in cases of doubt, proceed to angiography.

Intra-arterial drug administration
Intra-arterial drug administration leads to intense spasm and microvascular thrombosis. The leg is mottled and digital gangrene is common, but pedal pulses are usually palpable. The mainstay of treatment is supportive care, hydration to minimise renal failure secondary to rhabdomyolysis, and full heparinisation. Vascular reconstruction is almost never indicated, but fasciotomy may be required to prevent a compartment syndrome.

Venous gangrene
Venous gangrene can be mistaken for acute limb ischaemia. However, the leg is invariably swollen and the superficial veins full. Oedema may make it impossible to palpate pedal pulses, but Doppler examination will show normal distal waveforms and pressures. Management includes elevation, heparinisation, thrombolysis, and treatment of the underlying cause (usually pelvic or abdominal malignancy).

Aortic dissection
This may cause upper and lower limb ischaemia due to pinching of the ostia of the relevant arteries by the false lumen.

Thoracic outlet syndrome
Pressure on the subclavian artery from a cervical rib or abnormal soft tissue band may lead to a post-stenotic dilatation lined with thrombus, which predisposes to occlusion or

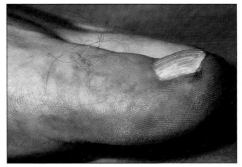
Blue toe syndrome must be promptly identified

Initial management of acute limb ischaemia
Sensation and movement absent
- Intravenous heparin
- Rapid resuscitation to best medical condition
- Intravenous fluids, catheter, and good urine output
- Urgent surgery—embolectomy or bypass

Sensation and movement present
- Optimise patient to best medical condition
- Admit to hospital
- Intravenous heparin
- Observe limb for signs of deterioration (and act if it occurs)
- Arteriogram when convenient

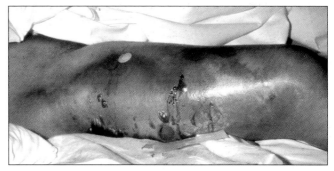
Compound fracture of tibia with ischaemia

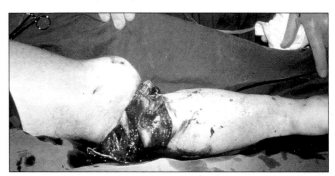
Ischaemia after intra-arterial drug administration

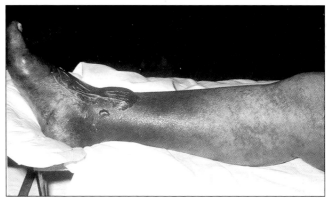
Venous gangrene

embolisation. The distal circulation may be chronically obliterated and digital ischaemia advanced before the thoracic outlet syndrome is diagnosed. The diagnosis is based on the results of duplex ultrasonography or angiography, or both. Treatment options include thrombolysis, thrombectomy or embolectomy, excision of the cervical rib, and repair of the aneurysmal segment.

Thrombolysis
In thrombolysis a cannula is embedded into the distal extent of the thrombus and streptokinase or, preferably, recombinant tissue plasminogen activator is infused. The technique cannot be used in patients with complete ischaemia because thrombus dissolution takes several hours. It is also relatively ineffective against the organised thrombus present in most peripheral emboli and is associated with an appreciable minor (20%, mainly groin haematoma) and major (5%, serious haemorrhage and stroke) complication rate. Thrombolysis should be undertaken only in an environment where experienced nursing and medical staff can closely monitor the patient.

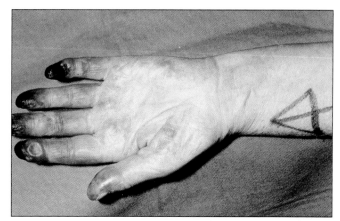
Digital gangrene due to pressure on subclavian artery from cervical rib

Post-ischaemic syndromes

Reperfusion injury
The reintroduction of oxygenated blood after a period of ischaemia causes more damage than the ischaemia alone. Generation of highly reactive, oxygen free radicals is greatly increased, and these activate neutrophils which migrate into the reperfused tissue causing injury. For vascular injury to occur neutrophils must be present and must adhere to the endothelium. The damaged endothelial cells become more permeable.

Effects of reperfusion syndrome
Local—Limb swelling due to increased capillary permeability causes a compartment syndrome, impaired muscle function due to ischaemia, and subsequent muscle contracture if the muscle infarcts.

General—Acidosis and hyperkalaemia occur due to leakage from the damaged cells, causing cardiac arrhythmias and myoglobinaemia, which can result in acute tubular necrosis. Acute respiratory distress syndrome may also develop, and gastrointestinal endothelial oedema may lead to increased gastrointestinal vascular permeability and endotoxic shock.

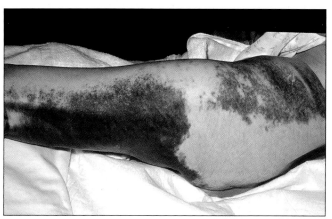
Haematoma due to thrombolysis

Compartment syndrome
Increased capillary permeability and oedema on reperfusion in the calf, where muscles are confined within tight fascial boundaries, causes an increase in interstitial pressure leading to muscle necrosis despite apparently adequate inflow—compartment syndrome. There is swelling and pain on squeezing the calf muscle or moving the ankle. Palpable pedal pulses do not exclude the syndrome. The key to management is prevention through expeditious revascularisation and a low threshold for fasciotomy. (If in doubt—do it.)

Chronic pain syndromes
Acute complete ischaemia can lead to peripheral nerve injury that manifests as the chronic pain syndrome, also referred to as causalgia, reflex sympathetic dystrophy, and many other terms. If the syndrome is recognised and treated early then many patients gain prolonged relief from drugs or chemical or surgical sympathectomy.

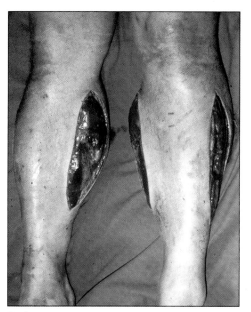
Fasciotomy

We thank Professor C V Ruckley, Mr A Jenkins, and Mr J A Murie for help with the illustrations.

3 Chronic lower limb ischaemia

Jonathan D Beard

Peripheral vascular disease commonly affects the arteries supplying the leg and is mostly caused by atherosclerosis. Restriction of blood flow, due to arterial stenosis or occlusion, often leads patients to complain of muscle pain on walking (intermittent claudication). Any further reduction in blood flow causes ischaemic pain at rest, which affects the foot. Ulceration and gangrene may then supervene and can result in loss of the limb if not treated. The Fontaine score is useful when classifying the severity of ischaemia.

Although many patients with claudication remain stable, about 150-200 per million of the population progress to critical limb ischaemia (Fontaine III or IV) each year. Many patients with critical limb ischaemia can undergo revascularisation, which has a reasonable chance of saving the limb. A recent audit by the Vascular Surgical Society found a success rate of over 70% for these patients. However, many patients still require major amputation. Rehabilitation of elderly patients after amputation can prove difficult, with high community costs. Critical limb ischaemia has been estimated to cost over £200m a year in the United Kingdom.

Intermittent claudication

History and examination

A history of muscular, cramp-like pain on walking that is rapidly relieved by resting, together with absent pulses, strongly supports the diagnosis of intermittent claudication. Disease of the superficial femoral artery in the thigh results in absent popliteal and foot pulses and often causes calf claudication. Disease of the aorta or iliac artery results in a weak or absent femoral pulse, often associated with a femoral bruit. Disease at this level may cause calf, thigh, or buttock claudication.

Fontaine classification of chronic leg ischaemia

Stage I Asymptomatic
Stage II Intermittent claudication
Stage III Ischaemic rest pain
Stage IV Ulceration or gangrene, or both

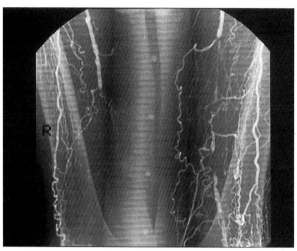

Angiogram showing bilateral occlusions of superficial femoral arteries in thighs. Collaterals arising from the profunda femoris artery can functionally bypass this occlusion

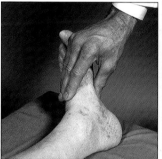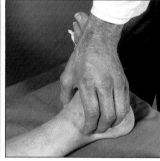

Method of palpating dorsalis pedis (left) and posterior tibial (right) pulses. Examine pulses from the foot of the bed, keeping the fingers flat for the dorsalis pedis and using the fingertips for the posterior tibial, while applying counterpressure with the thumb

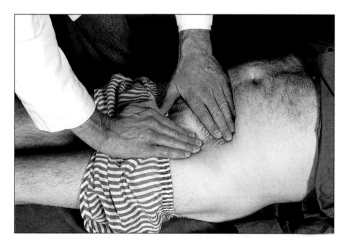

Method of palpating femoral pulse in skin crease of groin. Counterpressure on the lower abdomen pushes the skin crease towards the inguinal ligament and reduces the risk of missing the pulse

The dorsalis pedis artery lies superficially on the dorsum of the foot, although its position varies considerably. The posterior tibial artery lies deeper behind the medial malleolus. Many healthy people have only one foot pulse. The popliteal pulse can be difficult to palpate in muscular patients. A prominent popliteal pulse suggests the possibility of a popliteal aneurysm.

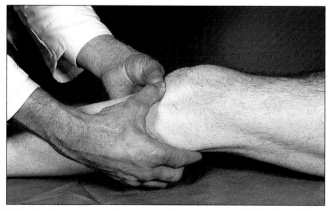

Method of palpating popliteal artery with patient's knee slightly flexed. Use thumbs to apply counterpressure while palpating the artery, which lies deep in popliteal fossa, with fingers

Differential diagnosis

The pain of nerve root compression can be mistaken for vascular claudication. A careful history can usually distinguish nerve root compression, especially sciatica due to compression of the lumbosacral root. However, compression of the cauda equina due to spinal stenosis can be more difficult to diagnose. This condition usually causes pain that radiates down both legs. Although the pain is made worse by walking, it also comes on after prolonged standing and is not rapidly relieved by rest, unlike vascular claudication.

Investigation

There are many causes of leg pain that can occur in the presence of asymptomatic peripheral vascular disease. Therefore, the absence of pulses does not necessarily imply a causal link. Furthermore, the presence of pulses at rest does not exclude symptomatic peripheral vascular disease. A good history together with an ankle brachial systolic pressure index of less than 0.9 confirms the diagnosis.

Exercise testing provides an objective measurement of walking distance, and highlights other exercise limiting conditions such as arthritis and breathlessness. However, exercise testing takes time, and many patients find it difficult or impossible to walk on a treadmill. Only those with a good history of claudication and normal resting ankle brachial systolic pressure indexes require an exercise test.

Duplex ultrasound scanning is useful for delineating the anatomical site of disease in the lower limb. Many hospitals still use arteriography for this purpose or when the results of duplex scanning are equivocal. This invasive and expensive investigation should not be requested unless there is a plan to proceed with revascularisation, if possible.

Principles of treatment

Intermittent claudication seems a relatively benign condition, although severe claudication may preclude patients from manual work. The risk of generalised vascular disease is probably more important. Patients with claudication have a three times higher risk of death compared with age matched controls. Modification of risk factors is therefore vital to reduce death from myocardial infarction and stroke. All patients should be advised to stop smoking and take regular exercise. They should also be screened for hyperlipidaemia and diabetes. Patients with peripheral vascular disease benefit from regular chiropody, and those with diabetes should attend a foot clinic. Obesity reduces exercise capacity, and losing weight will improve the walking distance.

Drug treatment

All patients with peripheral vascular disease benefit from aspirin (75-300 mg/day) because this reduces the risk of cardiovascular events. Patients who are intolerant of aspirin should take dipyridamole (200 mg, twice daily) or clopidogrel (75 mg/day). Naftidrofuryl may improve the walking distance of patients with moderate claudication (less than 500 m), but it is not known if it affects the outcome of the disease. The evidence to support naftidrofuryl is controversial, and patients prescribed it should be reassessed after three to six months.

Exercise programmes

A recent meta-analysis of 21 supervised exercise programmes showed that training for at least six months, by walking to near maximum pain tolerance, significantly improved pain free and maximum walking distances. The only controlled trial comparing an exercise programme with percutaneous transluminal angioplasty found that exercise was better. Exercise programmes are cheaper than percutaneous

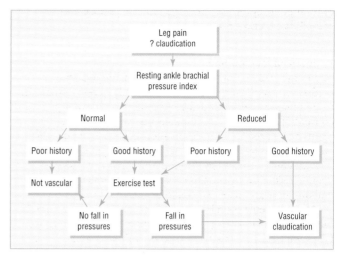

Algorithm for investigation of suspected intermittent claudication

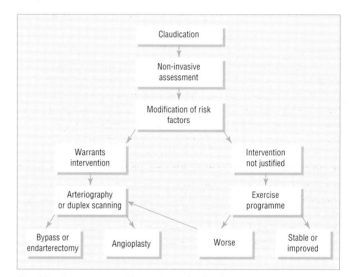

Algorithm for treatment of intermittent claudication

Factors which may influence the decision to treat claudication

For	Against
Severe symptoms	Short history
Job affected	Continued smoking
No better after exercise training	Severe angina or chronic obstructive airways disease
Stenosis or short occlusion	Long occlusion
Proximal disease	Distal disease
Unilateral disease	Multilevel disease

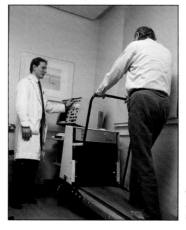

Treadmills can be used for objective measurement of walking distance and for exercise training

transluminal angioplasty or surgery, although long term compliance seems poor.

Endovascular techniques
The number of percutaneous transluminal angioplasties performed for claudication has risen steeply in recent years. In some situations endovascular techniques have virtually replaced conventional surgery. Percutaneous transluminal angioplasty seems best suited for stenoses or short occlusions of the iliac and superficial femoral vessels, with one year patency rates of 90% and 80% respectively. Angioplasty carries a small but definite risk of losing the limb because of thrombosis or embolisation, and patients should be informed of this risk.

Metallic stents push back the atheroma and improve on the initial lumen gain after angioplasty alone. The indications for iliac stents include a residual stenosis or dissection after angioplasty and long occlusions, but there seems little evidence to justify their routine use. Deployment of stents more distally has produced disappointing results due to high restenosis rates.

Surgery
The role of bypass for longer arterial occlusions remains poorly defined because of a lack of proper trials comparing it with percutaneous transluminal angioplasty and conservative treatment. Polyester (Dacron) aortobifemoral bypass grafts have five year patency rates of over 90% but are associated with a mortality of up to 5%. Complications include graft infection and postoperative impotence. Femoropopliteal bypass grafting, using autologous long saphenous vein, polyester, or polytetrafluoroethylene (Goretex) yields patency rates of less than 70% at five years. The early patency of prosthetic grafts seems similar to that of vein grafts, although the long term results seem less good. Femoropopliteal bypass grafts should rarely be used for patients with claudication.

Critical limb ischaemia

History and examination
Patients with critical limb ischaemia often describe a history of deteriorating claudication, progressing to nocturnal rest pain. Ulceration or gangrene commonly results from minor trauma. Nocturnal rest pain often occurs just after the patient has fallen asleep when the systemic blood pressure falls, further reducing perfusion to the foot. Hanging the foot out of bed increases perfusion and produces the typical dusky red hue due to loss of capillary tone. Elevation causes pallor and venous guttering. Inspect the foot carefully for ulceration under the heel and between the toes. Swelling suggests deep infection. If you can palpate foot pulses consider an alternative cause of pain, such as gout. Patients with critical limb ischaemia require urgent referral to a vascular surgeon.

Investigation
The ankle brachial systolic pressure index is usually less than 0.5. Arterial calcification may result in falsely increased pressures, and caution is needed when relying on Doppler pressures alone, especially in diabetic patients. All patients with critical limb ischaemia should ideally have arteriography with a view to endovascular treatment, if feasible. Duplex scanning may be used instead of angiography and for mapping of the long saphenous vein before distal bypass surgery. Dependent Doppler or pulse generated run-off can help to determine the most suitable artery to receive a distal bypass graft if these cannot be identified by angiography.

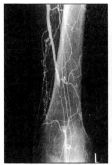
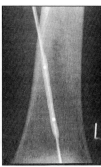
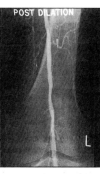

Short occlusion of left popliteal artery (left) treated by percutaneous transluminal angioplasty. The balloon catheter is passed through the occlusion over a guide wire and inflated (middle). Appearance after angioplasty is shown on right

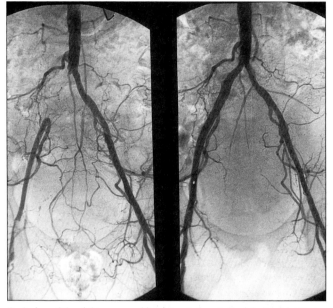

Occlusion of the right common iliac artery before (left) and after (right) insertion of stent

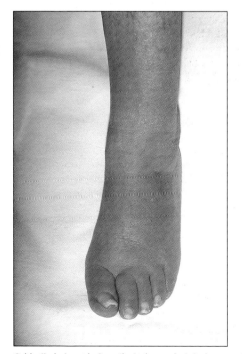

Critically ischaemic foot displaying typical dusky red hue on dependency (ischaemic rubor)

Principles of treatment

The same principles and techniques used to treat claudication also apply to critical limb ischaemia. However, critical limb ischaemia is usually caused by multilevel disease, which means that success rates are lower. Treatment focuses on saving the limb, although modification of risk factors remains important.

Endovascular treatment

Percutaneous transluminal angioplasty or stenting of proximal disease may relieve ischaemic rest pain, but healing of ulceration or gangrene usually requires restoration of foot pulses. This may necessitate extensive angioplasty of the superficial femoral, popliteal, and tibial arteries. Good results have been reported with subintimal angioplasty. Endovascular treatment can also reduce the magnitude of subsequent surgery.

Surgery

Patients with a pattern of arterial disease considered unsuitable for endovascular treatment will usually require surgery. Fit patients with proximal disease benefit greatly from aortobifemoral bypass grafting. In unfit patients the options include crossfemoral bypass for unilateral disease or axillobifemoral bypass for bilateral disease. These extra-anatomic procedures have lower patency rates. Many patients with distal disease will require bypass grafting to the popliteal or crural arteries below the knee. Autologous vein grafts give the best patency rates (70% at one year). Postoperative duplex surveillance may improve patency by permitting the detection and treatment of vein graft stenoses before occlusion occurs.

Amputation

Patients with unreconstructable peripheral vascular disease, fixed flexion deformities, or extensive tissue loss usually require a major amputation. Preservation of the knee joint has enormous advantages for wearing artificial limbs and subsequent mobility. However, there is little point in risking a non-healing, below knee amputation if the patient seems unlikely to walk again. Similarly, a patient with good prospects of wearing an artificial limb will fare better with an above knee amputation, if below knee amputation seems unachievable. Local amputation of ulcerated or gangrenous toes will not heal without revascularisation.

Pain relief

Critical limb ischaemia causes severe pain that requires narcotic analgesia to provide relief. A slow release opiate such as morphine seems a good option. Opiates can be supplemented by non-steroidal anti-inflammatory drugs if these are not contraindicated. Apart from rehydration, adequate analgesia alone may be the best treatment for patients with dementia or other severe comorbidity. If opiate analgesia remains inadequate, then lumbar sympathectomy (surgical or chemical) or spinal cord stimulation may help.

About 20-30% of patients with critical limb ischaemia have unreconstructable disease. A meta-analysis of six randomised trials of Iloprost, a stable prostacyclin analogue, found that infusion of this drug reduced the death and amputation rate. Phantom limb pain may complicate major amputation. Amitryptyline, carbamazepine, transcutaneous nerve stimulation, and acupuncture can help in this situation.

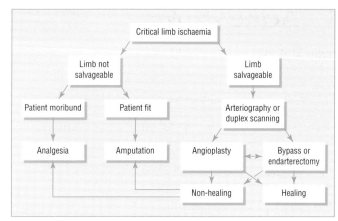

Algorithm for treatment of critical limb ischaemia

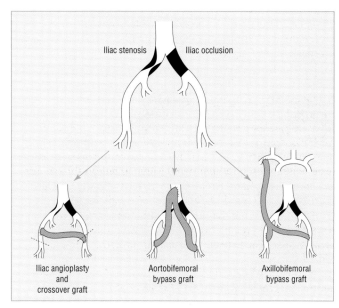

Surgical treatment options for aortoiliac disease

Methods of pain relief for critical limb ischaemia

- Slow release opiate analgesia—for example, morphine sulphate
- Prostacyclin analogues*—for example, Iloprost or prostaglandin E_1 (alprostadil)
- Chemical or surgical lumbar sympathectomy
- Dorsal column spinal stimulation

*Not licensed in United Kingdom

Further reading

- Scottish Intercollegiate Guidelines Network. Drug therapy for peripheral vascular disease. *SIGN* 1998;27.
- Joint British recommendations on the prevention of coronary heart disease in clinical practice. *Heart* 1998;80(suppl):S1-29.
- Leng GC, Fowler B, Ernst F. Exercise for intermittent claudication. In: *Cochrane Library*. Issue 4. Oxford: Update Software, 1999.
- Davies AH, Beard JD, Wyatt MG. *Essential vascular surgery*. London; W B Saunders, 1999.

4   Acute stroke

Philip M W Bath, Kennedy R Lees

Acute stroke is now a treatable condition that deserves urgent specialist attention. Drug treatment and specialist care both influence survival and recovery. This article considers the optimal approaches to diagnosis and early management.

Stroke, a sudden neurological deficit of presumed vascular origin, is a clinical syndrome rather than a single disease. It is a common and devastating condition that causes death in one third of patients at six months and leaves another third permanently dependent on the help of others. Each year in the United Kingdom there are 110 000 first strokes and 30 000 recurrent strokes; 10 000 strokes occur in people younger than 65 and 60 000 people die of stroke. It is the largest cause of disability, and more than five per cent of NHS and social services resources are consumed by stroke patients. Correct management relies on rapid diagnosis and treatment, thorough investigation, and rehabilitation.

Assessing the patient

Patients should be assessed at hospital immediately after a stroke. They may need to go straight to hospital rather than wait to see their general practitioner since hyperacute treatments such as thrombolysis must be administered within as little as three hours after stroke. Ambulance crews can be trained to apply simple screening questions to identify likely stroke patients.

Stroke is a clinical diagnosis, but brain imaging is required to distinguish ischaemia from primary intracerebral haemorrhage. The pattern of neurological signs, including evidence of motor, sensory, or cortical dysfunction and hemianopia, can be used to diagnose certain clinical subtypes and thus to predict prognosis. Other signs also relate to outcome and may help identify the cause. If neurological symptoms resolve in less than 24 hours, the traditional diagnostic label is "transient ischaemic attack" rather than stroke. However, not all transient ischaemic attacks are genuinely ischaemic, and many are associated with permanent cerebral damage: a better term therefore is "mini-stroke."

Pathophysiology

For practical purposes, there are two types of stroke after subarachnoid haemorrhage has been excluded. Ischaemia accounts for 85% of presentations and primary haemorrhage for 15%. Haemorrhage causes direct neuronal injury, and the pressure effect causes adjacent ischaemia. Primary ischaemia results from atherothrombotic occlusion or an embolism. The usual sources of embolism are the left atrium in patients with atrial fibrillation or the left ventricle in patients with myocardial infarction or heart failure.

Vessel occlusion arises from atherosclerosis, typically in the internal carotid artery just above the carotid bifurcation or from small vessel disease deep within the brain. Ischaemia causes direct injury from lack of oxygenation and nutritional support and sets up a cascade of neurochemical events that lead to spreading damage. The ischaemia may be reversible if reperfusion is obtained quickly (now proved in clinical trials), and the chemical injury may be interrupted by various neuroprotective drugs (unproved in humans).

Conditions requiring referral to hospital

Admit to hospital
- Neurological deficit lasting 1 hour or more
- Dependent patients—that is, moderate to severe stroke
- Transient ischaemic attack lasting 1 hour or more
- More than one transient ischaemic attack within a week
- Transient ischaemic attack on anticoagulation
- Patient presenting to hospital
- At request of general practitioner

Refer to cerebrovascular clinic
- Independent patient more than 48 hours after stroke (withhold aspirin)
- Transient ischaemic attack lasting less than 1 hour (give aspirin)

Symptoms and signs of stroke

Anterior circulation strokes
- Unilateral weakness
- Unilateral sensory loss or inattention
- Isolated dysarthria
- Dysphasia
- Vision:
  Homonymous hemianopia
  Monocular blindness
  Visual inattention

Posterior circulation strokes
- Isolated homonymous hemianopia
- Diplopia and disconjugate eyes
- Nausea and vomiting
- Incoordination and unsteadiness
- Unilateral or bilateral weakness and/or sensory loss

Non-specific signs
- Dysphagia
- Incontinence
- Loss of consciousness

Characteristics of subtypes of stroke

	Lacunar	Partial anterior circulation	Total anterior circulation	Posterior circulation
Signs	Motor or sensory only	2 of following: motor or sensory; cortical; hemianopia	All of: motor or sensory; cortical; hemianopia	Hemianopia; brain stem; cerebellar
% dead at 1 year	10	20	60	20
% dependent at 1 year	25	30	35	20

Signs of stroke at clinical examination

- Conscious level
- Neurological signs
- Blood pressure
- Heart rate and rhythm
- Heart murmurs
- Peripheral pulses
- Systemic signs of infection or neoplasm

Emergency management

Within the first hours after onset of cerebral ischaemia part of the brain is under threat of death. The infarct core may be densely ischaemic and will inevitably die, but there is also tissue with a compromised blood supply balanced on a knife edge between death and recovery. At this stage, oxygenation and haemodynamic and metabolic factors are crucial. The emergency management of stroke requires medical stabilisation and assessment of factors that may lead to complications (such as swallowing and hydration); thrombolysis may be considered (see below). An acute stroke unit concentrates patients, healthcare staff, resources, and expertise into one area, and such units may be associated with a better outcome.

Investigations

Patients with acute stroke should have computed tomography of the brain to distinguish ischaemic and haemorrhagic stroke. This separation is vital since subsequent investigations and treatment differ for the two types. Neuroimaging will also identify conditions mimicking stroke and can help predict outcome. Ideally, imaging will be performed soon after admission. Magnetic resonance imaging of the brain may eventually replace computed tomography since it not only identifies stroke anatomy but can also assess blood flow and perfusion in the brain, detect whether lesions are new or old, and identify carotid artery stenosis.

Death rate (percentage) 30 days, one year, and five years after different types of stroke

	30 days	1 year	5 years
Ischaemic stroke	10	23	52
Intracerebral haemorrhage	52	62	70
Subarachnoid haemorrhage	45	48	52

Conditions that mimic stroke

Diagnosis	Diagnostic features
Decompensation of previous stroke	Evidence of infection such as urinary or respiratory tract; metabolic disturbance
Cerebral neoplasm (primary or secondary)	Less abrupt onset; primary tumour or secondary to, for example, lung or breast cancer
Subdural haematoma	Recent head injury
Epileptic seizure	Possible previous episodes
Traumatic brain injury	History of trauma
Migraine	Less abrupt onset; followed by headache; younger patients
Multiple sclerosis	Less abrupt onset; possible previous episodes
Cerebral abscess	Infection

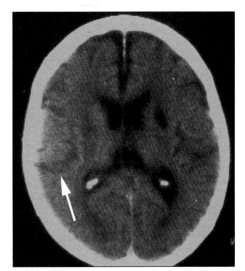

Computed tomogram showing ischaemic stroke

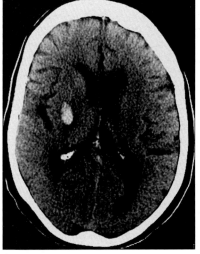

Computed tomogram showing haemorrhagic stroke

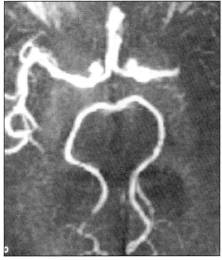

Magnetic resonance angiogram showing middle cerebral artery occlusion

The extent to which the cause of the stroke should be investigated depends on several factors, including the likely degree of recovery, the presence of obvious risk factors, and the age of the patient; younger patients are more likely to have an identifiable cause such as an inflammatory or clotting disorder which may require specific treatment. Although investigations should be restricted to tests that will inform clinical management, guidelines can be used to determine which investigations are needed after stroke.

Swallowing and feeding

Dysphagia affects 35% of stroke patients. It is often unrecognised after mild stroke and is associated with a poor outcome, partly because it predisposes to aspiration and pneumonia and partly because of the nutritional deficit. Presence of a gag reflex is a poor guide to safe swallowing, and a formal assessment by trained staff is essential. Fluids are more difficult to swallow than semisolids. Dysphagic patients should be fed through a nasogastric tube or percutaneous endoscopic

Investigation of stroke

All patients
- Computed tomography (or magnetic resonance imaging)
- Electrocardiography
- Chest radiography
- Full blood count
- Clotting screen
- Electrolyte and creatinine concentrations

Subgroups
- Carotid duplex scanning
- Echocardiography
- Thrombophilia screen
- Immunology screen
- Syphilis serology
- Cerebral angiography (rarely)

feeding tube until it is safe to resume oral food and fluids. Most dysphagic patients will not need enteral feeding beyond a few weeks. However, when and how optimally to feed dysphagic patients remains to be determined.

Acute intervention

Firm evidence from two large trials has shown that aspirin (160-300 mg daily by mouth, nasogastric tube, or rectum) started within 48 hours of onset of acute ischaemic stroke reduces the risk of subsequent death and disability. However, the effect of aspirin is small (number needed to treat (NNT) = 77) and is principally mediated through reducing the risk of early reinfarction. Neuroimaging is strongly recommended before starting aspirin. A large trial of unfractionated heparin in stroke patients found that heparin did not improve outcome, even in patients with presumed embolic stroke. Heparin may still be useful in certain groups of patients.

Thrombolysis with alteplase within three hours of onset of stroke significantly increases the chance of a near complete recovery (NNT = 7) when administered by specialists. Treatment up to six hours after stroke has been found less effective in meta-analysis of randomised controlled trials (estimated NNT = 12). Thrombolysis is currently licensed for stroke only in North America, and concerns remain about its safety.

Neuroprotectant drugs (which may protect neurones from ischaemia) have, to date, shown no benefit in ischaemic or haemorrhagic stroke, although several trials are still in progress.

Patients with a large cerebellar infarct or bleed should be referred for immediate neurosurgical evaluation to facilitate evacuation of the clot or infarct, or shunting for acute hydrocephalus, if required. Anticoagulants should be reversed in patients with primary intracerebral haemorrhage.

Complications of stroke

Stroke may be complicated by several conditions that can alter outcome adversely. Hyperglycaemia, fever, and hypertension are each associated with a poor prognosis. In the absence of trial evidence, raised glucose concentrations should be normalised and paracetamol given for fever. In contrast, hypertension should not be treated for the first week since some antihypertensive drugs (notably calcium channel blockers) seem to worsen outcome, possibly by reducing regional cerebral blood flow. Large ischaemic strokes are often complicated by oedema, swelling, and herniation leading to death; no proved treatment is available for these complications.

Venous thromboembolic disease (deep vein thrombosis, pulmonary embolism) develops in half of immobile patients unless preventive measures are taken. Although compression stockings reduce the risk of deep vein thrombosis in other groups of high risk patients, this has not been confirmed in stroke. A combination of stockings, early mobilisation, adequate hydration, and aspirin is considered good practice in patients with ischaemic stroke. Early mobilisation may also reduce the risk of pressure sores, respiratory tract infections, and urinary tract infections. When possible, urinary catheters should be avoided to minimise the risk of infection.

Rehabilitation

The principal aims of rehabilitation are to restore function and reduce the effect of the stroke on patients and their carers. Rehabilitation should start early during recovery with assessment and mobilisation while the patient is in the acute stroke unit. Once patients are medically stable, they should be

---

Acute drug treatments for ischaemic stroke

Aspirin
- Most patients

Heparin (unfractionated or low molecular weight):
Prophylactic
- Previous venous thromboembolism
- Morbid obesity

Therapeutic
- Carotid artery dissection
- Embolic, recurrent transient ischaemic attacks

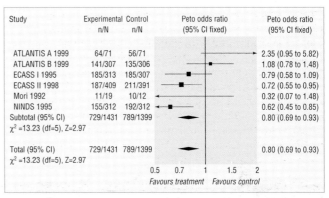

Study	Experimental n/N	Control n/N	Peto odds ratio (95% CI fixed)	Peto odds ratio (95% CI fixed)
ATLANTIS A 1999	64/71	56/71		2.35 (0.95 to 5.82)
ATLANTIS B 1999	141/307	135/306		1.08 (0.78 to 1.48)
ECASS I 1995	185/313	185/307		0.79 (0.58 to 1.09)
ECASS II 1998	187/409	211/391		0.72 (0.55 to 0.95)
Mori 1992	11/19	10/12		0.32 (0.07 to 1.48)
NINDS 1995	155/312	192/312		0.62 (0.45 to 0.85)
Subtotal (95% CI)	729/1431	789/1399		0.80 (0.69 to 0.93)
χ^2 =13.23 (df=5), Z=2.97				
Total (95% CI)	729/1431	789/1399		0.80 (0.69 to 0.93)
χ^2 =13.23 (df=5), Z=2.97				

0.5   0.7   1   1.5   2
Favours treatment   Favours control

Meta-analysis shows that thrombolysis reduces combined death and disability from stroke

---

Complications of stroke
- Hyperglycaemia
- Hypertension
- Fever
- Infarct extension or rebleeding
- Cerebral oedema, herniation, coning
- Aspiration
- Pneumonia
- Urinary tract infection
- Cardiac dysrhythmia
- Recurrence
- Deep vein thrombosis, pulmonary embolism

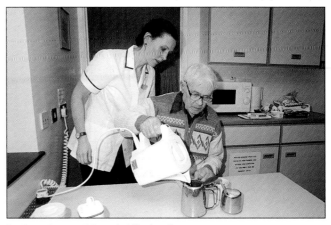

Stroke patient receiving rehabilitation therapy

transferred to a stroke rehabilitation unit if further rehabilitation is required. Formal rehabilitation in a stroke unit is associated with reduced death and disability (NNT = 12) and a shorter stay in hospital. Optimal care is multidisciplinary: doctors, nurses, physiotherapists, occupational therapists, speech and language therapists, dieticians, psychologists, and social workers all have a role.

Secondary prevention

Secondary prevention (apart from blood pressure control) should start shortly after admission. All patients should be offered lifestyle guidance, including advice to stop smoking, reduce saturated fat and salt consumption and alcohol intake, lose weight, and increase exercise. Aspirin started for the treatment of acute ischaemic stroke should be continued indefinitely for secondary prevention. The use of alternative or additional antithrombotic drugs (dipyridamole, clopidogrel, and warfarin), carotid endarterectomy, and management of hypertension and hyperlipidaemia after stroke are discussed in the next article in the series.

The future

Stroke management is now supported by good quality evidence, but many questions remain unanswered. Whenever possible, patients should be given the opportunity to enrol in randomised trials of acute interventions, rehabilitation, or secondary prevention.

Healthcare professionals, patients, and carers can obtain further information about strokes from the Stroke Association (020 7566 0300), Chest, Heart and Stroke Association Scotland (0131 225 6963), Chest, Heart, and Stroke Association Northern Ireland (01232 320184), or Different Strokes (01908 236033)

Further reading
- Bath PMW. The medical management of stroke. *Int J Clin Pract* 1997;51:504-10.
- Lees KR. If I had a stroke.... *Lancet* 1998;352 (suppl III):28-30.
- Royal College of Physicians. *Stroke audit package*. London: RCP, 1994.
- Stroke Units Trialists' Collaboration. Collaborative systematic review of the randomised trials of organised inpatient (stroke unit) care after stroke. *BMJ* 1997;314:1151-9.

The magnetic resonance image was provided by Professor Alan Moody, University of Nottingham. The data on thrombolysis were provided by Dr Joanna Wardlaw, University of Edinburgh.

5 Secondary prevention of transient ischaemic attack and stroke

Kennedy R Lees, Philip M W Bath, A Ross Naylor

Stroke or transient ischaemic attack is common and likely to be fatal or cause serious disability. A second stroke will not necessarily be of the same type as the initial event, although haemorrhages tend to recur. Patients with previous stroke commonly succumb to other vascular events, in particular myocardial infarction. Effective secondary prevention depends on giving attention to all modifiable risk factors for stroke as well as treating the causes of the initial stroke. Four questions should be answered:

Is it acute cerebrovascular disease?

The key features of acute cerebrovascular disease are focal neurological deficit, sudden onset, and absence of an alternative explanation. Abrupt onset of a dense hemiparesis before gradual improvement in a conscious patient rarely causes doubt, but conditions which commonly mimic stroke must be considered (see previous article *BMJ* 2000;320:920-3).

Is it ischaemic or haemorrhagic stroke?

Neither clinical history nor examination can reliably distinguish infarction from primary intracerebral haemorrhage. A small bleed can produce transient symptoms, although these rarely resolve within an hour.

Cerebral imaging is essential, and the choice and timing of the scan is important. Haemorrhage is immediately apparent on computed tomography, but its distinctive appearance becomes indistinguishable from infarction over a few weeks; for major symptoms, a computed tomogram taken within two weeks should still be diagnostic, but a small bleed may be missed after one week.

Magnetic resonance imaging has a greater sensitivity for brain stem, cerebellar, and small ischaemic strokes of the brain than computed tomography. It can also identify haemorrhagic stroke and remains diagnostic long after signs have become undetectable on computed tomography.

Risk of recurrence after stroke or transient ischaemic attack

Stroke
- 8% a year

Transient ischaemic attack
- 8% risk of stroke in first month
- 5% risk of stroke a year thereafter
- 5% risk of myocardial infarction a year

Modifiable risk factors for stroke
- Hypertension
- Smoking
- Diabetes mellitus
- Diet: high salt and fats, low potassium and vitamins
- Excess alcohol intake
- Morbid obesity
- Low physical exercise
- Low temperature
- Cholesterol concentration—at least in patients with coronary disease

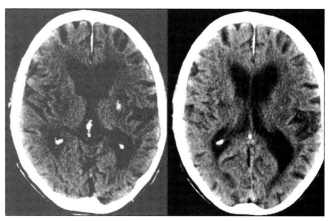

Computed tomograms on days 0 (left) and 8 (right) after left subcortical haemorrhage presenting as a transient ischaemic attack with symptoms lasting 50 minutes. Note the resolution of diagnostic appearances at day 8

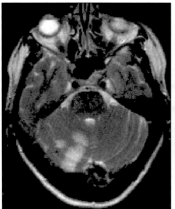

Magnetic resonance image of posterior fossa of brain in patient with right cerebellar infarction

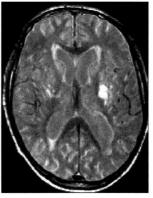

T1 weighted magnetic resonance image of left subcortical haemorrhage (day 9 in same patient as computed tomograms above)

Correct imaging techniques for patients with symptoms of stroke

	Symptoms for < 1 hour	Symptoms for > 1 hour; onset < 2 weeks	Symptoms for > 1 hour; onset > 2 weeks
Abrupt onset, typical cerebrovascular symptoms	Image only if anticoagulation proposed	Computed tomography	Magnetic resonance imaging
Insidious onset suspicious of tumour	Not applicable	Computed tomography with contrast	Computed tomography with contrast
Insidious onset suggestive of multiple sclerosis	Not applicable	Magnetic resonance imaging	Magnetic resonance imaging

Cardioembolic or vascular aetiology?

Up to a quarter of ischaemic strokes are due to embolism from the heart or major vessels. In these patients, full anticoagulation should be considered. Embolic stroke can affect any vascular territory but can rarely be diagnosed conclusively. Certain features should prompt a search for an embolic source. Transthoracic echocardiography is usually adequate, but transoesophageal echocardiography is justified if the results are equivocal or the index of suspicion is high.

Anterior or posterior circulation?

The vertebrobasilar arteries supply the brain stem, cerebellum, and occipital lobes; the cerebral hemispheres are supplied through the carotid arteries. This distinction is important since carotid Doppler ultrasonography with a view to endarterectomy is justified in patients with severe carotid disease only if symptoms have arisen from the anterior circulation.

Hospital referral

Although the approach to investigation of stroke is simple, few general practitioners will have open access to the necessary facilities or see sufficient cases to develop expertise in interpretation of the results. Patients with suspected stroke need urgent telephone or fax referral to a "fast track" specialist cerebrovascular clinic or stroke unit because of the time limitations on the diagnostic capability of computed tomography and the limited availability of magnetic resonance imaging.

Management of risk factors

Smoking is an important correctable risk factor and should be strongly discouraged. The risk of stroke of a smoker returns to that of a non-smoker within three to five years of stopping smoking.

Immediate reduction of blood pressure may be deleterious, but long term risk is inversely related to the blood pressure achieved. Treatment may therefore be justified even in patients with "normal" blood pressures. Hypertension should be treated one to two weeks after a stroke on the basis of British Hypertension Society guidelines. Patients at high risk of a further stroke (such as elderly people) derive the greatest benefit from treatment.

The role of serum cholesterol concentration in the pathogenesis of stroke remains debatable. Nevertheless, statins have been shown to reduce the risk of stroke in clinical trials of patients with coronary heart disease. Lowering cholesterol concentrations with a statin after atherosclerotic stroke or transient ischaemic attack probably reduces recurrent events and the risk of developing ischaemic heart disease. Since stroke patients represent such a high risk population, the cost of treatment may be justified.

Diabetes confers a substantial disadvantage for survival and functional outcome on patients with acute stroke. The mechanism for this is unknown, but since it is a long term effect, attempts should be made to normalise blood glucose concentrations. Blood pressure targets are lower for diabetic than non-diabetic patients.

Raised plasma homocysteine concentration is increasingly linked to premature vascular disease and can be easily lowered through vitamin supplements (folate and pyridoxine). Although the value of lowering homocysteine concentrations has not been proved, younger patients with raised plasma homocysteine concentrations may benefit.

Embolic causes of stroke found on echocardiography

- Mitral stenosis
- Left atrial enlargement (>4 cm)
- Dyskinetic or akinetic left ventricle
- Severe global left ventricular dysfunction
- Valvular vegetation
- Left atrial or ventricular thrombus
- Mitral valve calcification
- Calcific aortic valves or stenosis predispose to embolism but may not justify anticoagulation

---

Justifications for echocardiography

- Atrial fibrillation
- Heart failure
- Myocardial infarction within 3 months
- Electrocardiographic abnormalities:
    Myocardial infarction or ischaemia
    Bundle branch block
- Cardiac murmur
- Peripheral embolism
- Clinical events in ≥ 2 territories:
    Right and left hemisphere
    Anterior and posterior circulation
- ≥ 2 cortical events (even in same territory) unless severe ipsilateral carotid disease

---

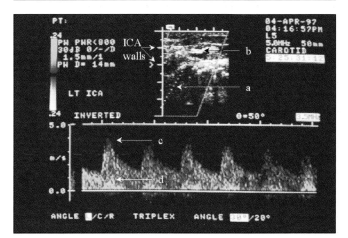

Carotid Doppler ultrasonogram in patient with severe internal carotid artery stenosis. Upper panel shows angle of insonation (a) of internal carotid artery and sampling window (b); the velocity of systolic blood flow at the point of maximal narrowing (c), is nearly 4 m/s (normal <1 m/s). Stenosis causes flow velocity to increase and produces turbulence, which is seen as shading within the Doppler spectrum (d)

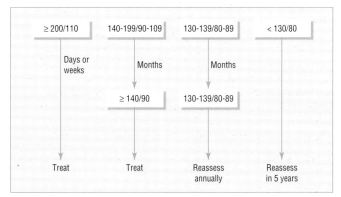

Blood pressure thresholds (mm Hg) for treatment after stroke or transient ischaemic attack (based on British Hypertension Society Guidelines 1999)

Blood pressure targets (mm Hg) in non-diabetic and diabetic stroke patients

	No diabetes	Diabetes
Titrate to diastolic blood pressure	≤ 85	≤ 80
Optimal blood pressure	$<140/85$	$<130/80$
Suboptimal blood pressure	$\geq 150/90$	$\geq 140/85$

Antiplatelet therapy and anticoagulation

Patients with atrial fibrillation should receive warfarin if they have no contraindications, aiming at an international normalised ratio of 2.0-3.0. Patients with other important sources of cardiac embolism also benefit from warfarin. Only patients with mechanical prosthetic heart valves require a higher international normalised ratio target of 2.5-4.5, although the exact value depends on the type of valve.

For all other patients with ischaemic stroke, antiplatelet therapy would be first line treatment. Aspirin is inexpensive and simple to administer, and its benefits are conclusively proved. An initial dose of 300 mg followed by 75 mg daily is advised (higher doses have little advantage but increase gastrointestinal side effects and bleeding).

Modified release dipyridamole (200 mg twice daily) has an independent and additive effect to low dose aspirin in preventing further strokes but not coronary events or overall mortality. The routine addition of dipyridamole to aspirin for secondary prevention of strokes may be cost effective.

Clopidogrel (75 mg daily), a new antiplatelet drug, is well tolerated and was slightly more effective than aspirin in a large trial. However, it is not cost effective for initial treatment. Clopidogrel should be used in patients with true intolerance to aspirin (allergy or intractable side effects on low dose enteric coated aspirin with or without antiulcer drugs); dipyridamole alone does not prevent cardiac events.

Carotid surgery and angioplasty

Firm evidence from two large trials has clarified the role of carotid endarterectomy in patients with ipsilateral severe carotid stenosis. Patients with severe disease benefit from surgery for up to 12 months after the most recent cerebral event. The benefit derived is inextricably linked to the operative risk (stroke or death within 30 days). In the randomised trials, the operative mortality in patients with severe disease was 1.0%, the risk of death or disabling stroke <4%, and the risk of death or any stroke <7.5%. Surgical risk is inversely proportional to surgical volume, implying that patients should be referred to busy carotid endarterectomy centres. Surgeons must quote their own risks rather than results obtained in trials.

Any patient presenting with carotid territory symptoms should be considered a potential candidate for carotid endarterectomy, and carotid Doppler ultrasonography should be done if the patient is fit for surgery. The presence or absence of a carotid bruit is irrelevant. An ongoing meta-analysis may further refine the indications, particularly regarding the management of women and patients with isolated retinal symptoms, who seem to have a lower overall risk of stroke.

Indications for carotid endarterectomy

Surgery not indicated
- Carotid territory symptoms and an ipsilateral 0-69% stenosis
- Complete occlusion of the carotid artery

Surgery indicated
- Carotid territory symptoms within 6 months and an ipsilateral 70-99% stenosis
- Carotid territory symptoms within 12 months and an ipsilateral 80-99% stenosis

---

A successful carotid endarterectomy is not a major procedure, and most patients can be discharged home the day after surgery. Neither clinical nor ultrasonographic surveillance

---

Main contraindications to long term warfarin treatment
- Gastrointestinal bleeding
- Active peptic ulceration
- Frequent falls
- Alcohol misuse
- History of intracranial haemorrhage
Age, by itself, is not a contraindication

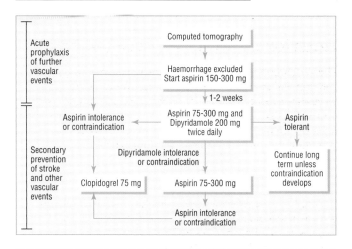

Summary of results from European carotid surgery trial

Stenosis (%)	Incidence of stroke (%)		Absolute risk reduction (%)	Relative risk reduction (%)
	Surgery arm	Medical arm		
0-30	11.8	6.2	−5.6 at 3 years	None
31-69	16.0	15.0	−1.0 at 5 years	None
70-99	12.3	21.9	9.6 at 3 years	44 at 3 years

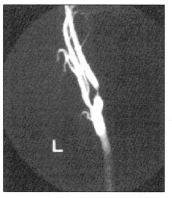

Angiogram showing tight stenosis of internal carotid artery just distal to bifurcation

---

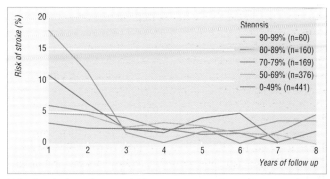

Risk of stroke in patients not having surgery according to degree of stenosis. Data from European Carotid Surgery Trialists' Collaborative Group, *Lancet* 1998;351:1379-87

prevents late stroke, and so most patients are discharged from follow up at six weeks with the proviso that they should be referred immediately should further cerebral ischaemic events occur.

In carotid angioplasty the stenosis is dilated by using a balloon catheter introduced percutaneously through the femoral artery. The potential advantages of carotid angioplasty include reduced hospital stay, cranial nerve injury, wound complications, and other cardiovascular morbidity. The main concern about carotid angioplasty is the risk of embolic stroke at the time of the procedure and recurrent stenosis. Carotid angioplasty aids the management of fibromuscular dysplasia, radiation injury, and symptomatic restenosis after carotid endarterectomy. Otherwise, carotid angioplasty should not be performed outside randomised trials and, as with carotid endarterectomy, outcomes in individual centres should be audited.

Complex cases

Secondary prevention of stroke is rightly the province of general practitioners and the preceding suggestions will cover most patients with recent stroke. However, patients with complex conditions will need access to specialist services, although definitive trial evidence justifying therapeutic decisions in such cases is often absent. Patients should be monitored for compliance with treatment and the development of complications such as renovascular disease, ischaemic heart disease, and further cerebrovascular problems. Optimal dietary, smoking, lipid, and blood pressure management is always required in addition to antithrombotic treatment.

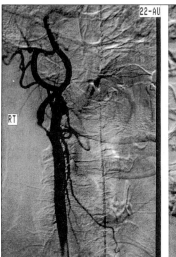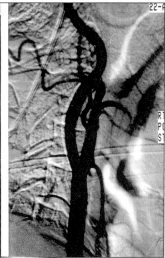

Severe carotid stenosis before (left) and after carotid angioplasty and stenting (right)

Complex cases that may require hospital referral

Case	Possible treatment
Recurrent stroke or transient ischaemic attack despite antiplatelet treatment (treatment failure)	Consider higher doses of aspirin, addition of dipyridamole (if not already prescribed), substitution or addition of clopidogrel, or substitution or addition of warfarin
Recurrent embolic events despite adequate anticoagulation with warfarin	Consider adding low dose aspirin
Recurrent non-haemodynamic symptoms from inoperable severe carotid stenosis or serious intracranial stenosis despite antiplatelet treatment	Consider warfarin
Hypertension and inoperable severe carotid stenosis	Consider cerebral blood flow monitoring (with ultrasonography or radionucleotide perfusion scanning) before antihypertensive treatment

Further reading

- Antiplatelet Trialists' Collaboration. Collaborative overview of randomised trials of antiplatelet therapy. 1. Prevention of death, myocardial infarction, and stroke by prolonged antiplatelet therapy in various categories of patients. *BMJ* 1994;308:81-106.
- EAFT (European Atrial Fibrillation Trial) Study Group. Secondary prevention in non-rheumatic atrial fibrillation after TIA or minor stroke. *Lancet* 1993;342:1255-62.
- Diener HC, Cunha L, Forbes C, Sivenius J, Smets P, Lowenthal A, for the ESPS-2 Working Group. European Stroke Prevention Study 2. Dipyridamole and acetylsalicylic acid in the secondary prevention of stroke. *J Neurol Sci* 1996;143:1-13.
- CAPRIE Steering Committee. A randomised, blinded, trial of clopidogrel versus aspirin in patients at risk of ischaemic events (CAPRIE). *Lancet* 1996;348:1329-39.
- European Carotid Surgery Trialists' Collaborative Group. Randomised trial of endarterectomy for recently symptomatic carotid stenosis. Final results of the MRC European carotid surgery trial (ECST). *Lancet* 1998;351:1379-87.

G T McInnes and L Ramsay contributed towards the blood pressure guidelines. M R Walters supplied some of the pictures and J Overell supplied the antiplatelet flow chart.

6 Vascular complications of diabetes

Richard Donnelly, Alistair M Emslie-Smith, Iain D Gardner, Andrew D Morris

Adults with diabetes have an annual mortality of about 5.4% (double the rate for non-diabetic adults), and their life expectancy is decreased on average by 5-10 years. Although the increased death rate is mainly due to cardiovascular disease, deaths from non-cardiovascular causes are also increased. A diagnosis of diabetes immediately increases the risk of developing various clinical complications that are largely irreversible and due to microvascular or macrovascular disease. Duration of diabetes is an important factor in the pathogenesis of complications, but other risk factors—for example, hypertension, cigarette smoking, and hypercholesterolaemia—interact with diabetes to affect the clinical course of microangiopathy and macroangiopathy.

Microvascular complications

A continuous relation exists between glycaemic control and the incidence and progression of microvascular complications. Hypertension and smoking also have an adverse effect on microvascular outcomes. In the diabetes control and complications trial—a landmark study in type 1 diabetes—the number of clinically important microvascular endpoints was reduced by 34-76% in patients allocated to intensive insulin (that is, a 10% mean reduction in glycated haemoglobin (Hb_{A1c}) concentration from 8.0% to 7.2%). However, these patients also had more hypoglycaemic episodes. Similarly, in the UK prospective diabetes study of patients with type 2 diabetes, an intensive glucose control policy that lowered glycated haemoglobin concentrations by an average of 0.9% compared with conventional treatment (median Hb_{A1c} 7.0% v 7.9%) resulted in a 25% reduction in the overall microvascular complication rate. It was estimated that for every 1% reduction in Hb_{A1c} concentration there is a 35% reduction in microvascular disease.

Retinopathy

Diabetic retinopathy is a progressive disorder classified according to the presence of various clinical abnormalities. It is the commonest cause of blindness in people aged 30-69 years. Damage to the retina arises from a combination of microvascular leakage and microvascular occlusion; these changes can be visualised in detail by fluorescein angiography. A fifth of patients with newly discovered type 2 diabetes have retinopathy at the time of diagnosis. In type 1 diabetes, vision threatening retinopathy almost never occurs in the first five years after diagnosis or before puberty. After 15 years, however,

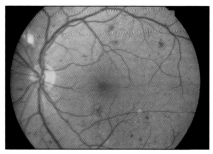

Background retinopathy showing microaneurysms and small blot haemorrhages

Risk of morbidity associated with all types of diabetes mellitus	
Complication	Relative risk*
Blindness	20
End stage renal disease	25
Amputation	40
Myocardial infarction	2-5
Stroke	2-3
*Compared with non-diabetic patients	

Vascular complications of diabetes

Microvascular	Macrovascular
Retinopathy	Ischaemic heart disease
Nephropathy	Stroke
Neuropathy	Peripheral vascular disease

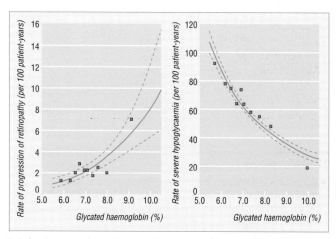

Relation between glycaemic control (Hb_{A1c}) and risk of progression of microvascular complications (retinopathy) and severe hypoglycaemia in patients with type 1 diabetes. Data from the diabetes control and complications trial. Dotted lines represent 95% confidence intervals

Classification and features of diabetic retinopathy

Grade	Examination features	Symptoms
I Background retinopathy	Microaneurysms Small blot haemorrhages Hard exudates Not affecting macula	None
II Background with maculopathy	Leakage in macular region Capillary occlusion Hard exudates	Central visual loss (such as reading difficulty)
III Preproliferative retinopathy	Cotton wool spots Venous abnormalities Large blot haemorrhages Intraretinal microvascular abnormalities	None
IV Proliferative retinopathy	New vessels on disc or elsewhere on retina	None, but complications cause visual loss
V Advanced diabetic eye disease	Extensive fibrovascular proliferation Retinal detachment Vitreous haemorrhage Thrombotic glaucoma	Severe visual loss

almost all patients with type 1 diabetes and two thirds of those with type 2 diabetes have background retinopathy.

Vision threatening retinopathy is usually due to neovascularisation in type 1 diabetes and maculopathy in type 2 diabetes. Depending on the relative contribution of leakage or capillary occlusion, maculopathy is divided into three types: exudative maculopathy (when hard exudates appear in the region of the macula), ischaemic maculopathy (characterised by a predominance of capillary occlusion which results in clusters of haemorrhages), and oedematous maculopathy (extensive leakage gives rise to macular oedema). Treatment of maculopathy and proliferative retinopathy with laser photocoagulation prevents further loss of vision rather than restores diminished visual acuity.

Nephropathy

Diabetic nephropathy is characterised by proteinuria >300 mg/24 h, increased blood pressure, and a progressive decline in renal function. At its most severe, diabetic nephropathy results in end stage renal disease requiring dialysis or transplantation, but in the early stages overt disease is preceded by a phase known as incipient nephropathy (or microalbuminuria), in which the urine contains trace quantities of protein (not detectable by traditional dipstick testing). Microalbuminuria is defined as an albumin excretion rate of 20-300 mg/24 h or 20-200 µg/min in a timed collection and is highly predictive of overt diabetic nephropathy, especially in type 1 diabetes.

The rate of decline in glomerular filtration rate varies widely between individuals, but antihypertensive treatment greatly slows the decline in renal function and improves survival in patients with diabetic nephropathy.

In patients with type 1 diabetes complicated by diabetic nephropathy, angiotensin converting enzyme inhibitors have renoprotective effects above those that can be attributed to reduced blood pressure; they are beneficial even in normotensive patients and ameliorate other associated microvascular complications such as retinopathy. In patients with type 2 diabetes, achieving good blood pressure control (which often requires combination therapy) is more important than the choice of antihypertensive drug, although angiotensin converting enzyme inhibitors are the preferred first line treatment

The development of proteinuria is a marker of widespread vascular damage and signifies an increased risk of subsequent end stage renal disease and macrovascular complications, especially coronary heart disease. Microproteinuria and proteinuria are strongly associated with decreased survival in both type 1 and type 2 diabetes.

Neuropathy

The diabetic neuropathies present in several ways. The commonest form is a diffuse progressive polyneuropathy affecting mainly the feet. It is predominantly sensory, often asymptomatic, and affects 40-50% of all patients with diabetes. Reduced sensation can be detected with a monofilament, and patients with sensory neuropathy as well as other high risk features need advice on foot care to minimise the risk of ulceration. Neuropathic foot ulcers can be distinguished from vascular ulcers, although a mixed aetiology is common.

Macrovascular complications

Atherosclerotic disease accounts for most of the excess mortality in patients with diabetes. In the UK prospective diabetes study, fatal cardiovascular events were 70 times more common than deaths from microvascular complications. The

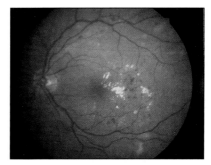

Diabetic maculopathy

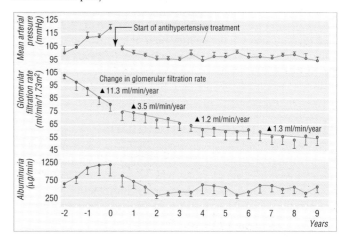

Effect of antihypertensive treatment (β blockers and diuretics) on mean arterial pressure, glomerular filtration rate, and albuminuria in patients with type 1 diabetes and nephropathy. Reproduced with permission from Mogensen, *Diabetic Med* 1995;12:756-9.

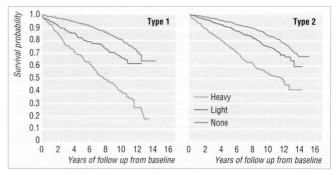

Data from WHO multinational study of vascular disease in diabetes showing survival in patients with type 1 and type 2 diabetes according to degree of proteinuria (none, slight, or heavy) at baseline. Reproduced with permission from Stephenson et al, *Diabetic Med* 1995;12:149-55

Clinical features of "high risk" diabetic foot

- Impaired sensation (monofilament)
- Past or current ulcer
- Maceration
- Fungal or gryphotic (thickened or horny) toenails
- Biomechanical problems (corns or callus)
- Fissures
- Clawed toes

Clinical features that distinguish neuropathic and vascular foot ulcers

Neuropathic	Vascular
Painless	Painful
Located at points of high pressure	Often located at the extremities
"Punched out" appearance surrounded by callus	
Warm foot	Cool ischaemic foot
Bounding foot pulses	Absent foot pulses

relation between glucose concentrations and macrovascular events is less powerful than for microvascular disease; smoking, blood pressure, proteinuria, and cholesterol concentration are more important risk factors for atheromatous large vessel disease in patients with diabetes.

Hyperlipidaemia is no more common in patients with well controlled type 1 diabetes than it is in the general population. In patients with type 2 diabetes, total and low density lipoprotein cholesterol concentrations are also similar to those found in non-diabetic people, but type 2 diabetes is associated with a more atherogenic lipid profile, in particular low concentrations of high density lipoprotein cholesterol and high concentrations of small, dense, low density lipoprotein particles.

Hypertension affects at least half of patients with diabetes. In the UK prospective diabetes study tight blood pressure control (mean 144/82 mm Hg) achieved significant reductions in the risk of stroke (44%), heart failure (56%), and diabetes related deaths (32%), as well as reductions in microvascular complications (for example, 34% reduction in progression of retinopathy). One third of patients required three or more antihypertensive drugs to maintain a target blood pressure < 150/85 mm Hg. In another recent study (hypertension optimal treatment study) rates of cardiovascular events in patients with type 2 diabetes were reduced even further when combination treatment was used to aim for target diastolic blood pressures < 80 mm Hg.

Coronary heart disease

The incidence and severity of coronary heart disease events are higher in patients with diabetes, and several clinical features are worth noting. The diabetes subgroups in the major secondary prevention studies of cholesterol reduction (Scandinavian

Predictors of cardiovascular mortality

Type 1 diabetes	Type 2 diabetes
● Overt nephropathy	● Presence of coronary heart disease
● Hypertension	● Overt proteinuria
● Smoking	● Glycated haemoglobin
● Microalbuminuria	● Hypertension
● Age	

Taken from *BMJ* 1996:313:779-84, *Diabetes*1995;44:1303-9

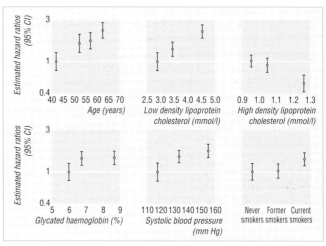

Estimated hazard ratios for significant risk factors for coronary heart disease occurring in 335 out of 3055 patients with type 2 diabetes. Reproduced from Turner et al, *BMJ* 1998;316:823-8.

Features of coronary heart disease in diabetic patients

Atherosclerosis
● Prevalence of fatal and non-fatal coronary heart disease events 2-20× higher than for non-diabetics of similar age
● Protective effect of female sex is lost
● Higher incidence of diffuse, multivessel disease
● Plaque rupture leading to unstable angina and myocardial infarction is more common
● Superimposed thrombosis more likely

Acute myocardial infarction
● In-hospital and 6 month mortality double that in non-diabetics
● Complications (eg, arrhythmias, heart failure, death) more common
● Reperfusion rates after thrombolysis are similar to those of non-diabetics, but reocclusion and reinfarction rates are higher
● Mortality reduced by insulin glucose infusion immediately after myocardial infarction

Revascularisation
● 5 year survival rates after coronary artery bypass graft or percutaneous coronary angioplasty lower than for non-diabetics
● 5 year survival better after coronary artery bypass graft than percutaneous coronary angioplasty because of higher restenosis rates with angioplasty (81% v 66%)

simvastatin survival study (4S) and cholesterol and recurrent events (CARE) trial) show a beneficial effect of statins.

Peripheral vascular disease

Atheromatous disease in the legs, as in the heart, tends to affect more distal vessels—for example, the tibial arteries—producing multiple, diffuse lesions that are less straightforward to bypass or dilate by angioplasty. Medial calcification of vessels (Mönckeberg's sclerosis) is common and can result in falsely raised measurements of the ankle brachial pressure index. This index is therefore less reliable as a screening test in patients with diabetes and intermittent claudication.

Stroke

Roughly 85% of acute strokes are atherothrombotic, and the rest are haemorrhagic (10% primary intracerebral haemorrhage and 5% subarachnoid haemorrhage). The risk of atherothrombotic stroke is two to three times higher in patients with diabetes, but the rates of haemorrhagic stroke and transient ischaemic attacks are similar to those of the non-diabetic population. Patients with

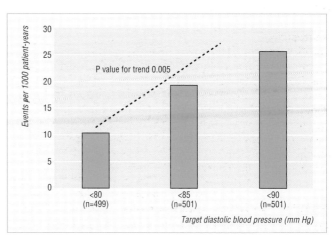

Rates of serious cardiovascular events according to target diastolic blood pressure in 1500 patients with hypertension and type 2 diabetes. Drawn from Hansson et al, *Lancet* 1998;351:1755-62.

diabetes are probably more prone to irreversible rather than reversible ischaemic brain damage, and small lacunar infarcts are common. Stroke patients with diabetes have a higher death rate and a poorer neurological outcome with more severe disability. Maintaining good glycaemic control immediately after a stroke is likely to improve outcome, but the long term survival is reduced because of a high rate of recurrence. Antihypertensive treatment is effective in preventing stroke.

Erectile dysfunction
Erectile dysfunction is a common complication of diabetes, occurring in up to half of men aged over 50 years (compared with 15-20% in age matched non-diabetic men), although the exact prevalance is unknown because of likely underreporting. The underlying pathogenesis is multifactorial, with autonomic neuropathy, vascular insufficiency, and psychological factors contributing to the clinical picture. The condition causes appreciable social and psychological problems for many patients, and its importance should not be underestimated. The recent introduction of sildenafil, which is reported to have a 50-70% success rate in patients with diabetes, is an important advance.

Surveillance and management in general practice
Screening for diabetes
Up to half of people with type 2 diabetes have vascular complications at the time of diagnosis. Early detection of diabetes is therefore essential. Screening (by measuring fasting blood glucose concentration) should be considered for high risk patients, especially those who are middle aged and obese, are of Asian or Afro-Caribbean origin, have a history of gestational diabetes, or have a family history of diabetes.

Eye screening
The small number of patients with retinopathy in any one practice (about 50 patients per 10 000 practice list) does not allow most general practitioners to develop and maintain their funduscopic skills. Innovative approaches, including the use of trained community optometrists and mobile retinal photography units that visit practices annually, can provide a high standard of retinal screening in the community.

Cardiovascular risk prediction
Identification of patients at highest risk of developing cardiovascular events allows efforts and resources to be channelled most effectively. Coronary risk prediction charts and computer programs such as that recently produced as

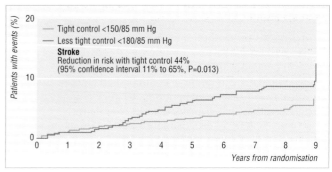

Kaplan-Meier plot of proportions of patients who developed fatal or non-fatal stroke, according to blood pressure control. Reproduced from Turner et al, *BMJ* 1998;317:703-13.

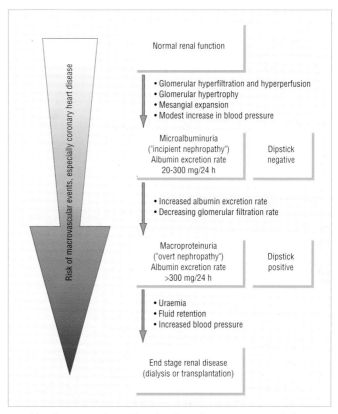

Transition from normal renal function through to end stage renal disease requiring dialysis or transplantation. Increasing proteinuria and renal impairment is associated with an increasing risk of fatal or non-fatal coronary heart disease, especially in older patients with type 2 diabetes and other risk factors

Recommendations on prevention of coronary heart disease in clinical practice

	Glycaemic control	Blood pressure control	Lipid control
Target	Glycated haemoglobin ≤7.0% Fasting blood glucose 4-7 mmol/l	≤140/80 mm Hg without macrovascular disease ≤130/80 mm Hg with macrovascular disease	Serum cholesterol <5.0 mmol/l in patients with established coronary heart disease Primary prevention in those with >30% risk of coronary heart disease over 10 years
Treatment (in addition to lifestyle and dietary advice)	Metformin (first line if body mass index >25) Sulphonylurea Acarbose Glitazones (not yet available in United Kingdom) Insulin Combination therapy	Angiotensin converting enzyme inhibitors: renoprotective but caution in renal artery stenosis (17% of hypertensive diabetics) Diuretics β blockers α blockers Long acting calcium antagonists 50% of patients will require ≥3 drugs for optimum control	Statins (regular monitoring of liver function)

Annual complications assessment

Physical examination
- Body mass index calculation (weight (kg)/(height (m))^2)
- Blood pressure measurement with patient sitting and appropriate sized cuff
- Palpation of foot pulses
- Measurement of foot sensation by one or more of following:
  10 g monofilament weight (not detected = impaired)
  Vibration of 128 Hz tuning fork over medial malleolus (perception for <5 secs = impaired)
  Assessment of ankle jerk with tendon hammer (less reliable in elderly people)
- Inspection of feet for nail care, callosities, fissures, fungal infection, blisters, ulcers, claw toes, prominent metatarsal heads, and Charcot arthropathy
- Visual acuity in corrected state, using standard 6 m (or 3 m) Snellen chart. Use pin hole if corrected acuity is ≥6/9
- Retinal examination by one of:
  Direct ophthalmoscopy through pupils dilated with 1% tropicamide
  Combination of direct ophthalmoscopy and slit lamp biomicroscopy
  Retinal photography through fixed site or mobile non-mydriatic fundus camera

Biochemical analysis
- Dipstick urine analysis for proteinuria
- Urine testing for microalbuminuria in type 1 diabetes
- Blood testing of:
  Glycated haemoglobin
  Serum creatinine
  Serum total cholesterol and high density lipoprotein cholesterol

History, advice, and education
- Smoking history
- Education and reinforcement of advice on diet, aerobic exercise, and lifestyle
- Review treatment, including side effects and compliance
- Assess knowledge of diabetes and self management skills, including warning signs for complications (intermittent claudication, angina pectoris, foot problems)
- Review footwear provision
- Review need for contact with dietetics, chiropody, orthotics, and diabetes specialist nurse support
- Advice on erectile dysfunction in men
- Prepregnancy counselling, where appropriate
- Calculate and discuss risk of coronary heart disease and modification of risk factors

---

part of the joint British recommendations on prevention of coronary heart disease in clinical practice will help general practitioners to implement the findings of recent major clinical trials.

Annual complications assessment
All patients with diabetes should be offered an annual clinical assessment concentrating on the prevention, detection, and management of macrovascular and microvascular complications.

Areas of debate in surveillance of diabetes complications
The value of routine measurements of microalbuminuria in patients with type 2 diabetes is less clear than in type 1 diabetes. Arrangements to allow the testing of microalbuminuria in general practice are not universally available.

The presence of left ventricular hypertrophy is a powerful predictor of the risk of a cardiovascular event, but screening by echocardiography or electrocardiography is often not included as part of the routine annual assessment.

Unlike total cholesterol concentrations and the total cholesterol to high density lipoprotein cholesterol ratio, the importance of raised triglyceride concentrations in the risk profile of patients with type 2 diabetes is unclear.

Team approach to integrated diabetic care
The ongoing care of patients with diabetes, in particular once they have developed vascular complications, includes a wide spectrum of healthcare professionals. A systematic, integrated, and collaborative approach must be developed at a regional level, with clear lines of communication and the adoption of locally agreed guidelines for treatment and referral based on national guidelines—for example, those from the Scottish Intercollegiate Guideline Network (www.show.scot.nhs.UK/sign/home.htm).

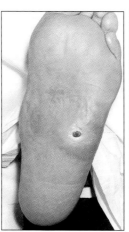

Neuropathic ulcer is a common complication in patients with diabetes

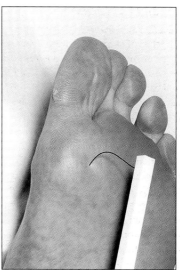

Use of monofilament to detect impaired sensation during annual assessment

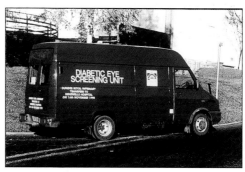

Mobile eye screening unit

7   Renal artery stenosis

Kevin McLaughlin, Alan G Jardine, Jon G Moss

Renal artery stenosis is becoming increasingly common because of atherosclerosis in an ageing population. Patients usually present with hypertension and varying degrees of renal impairment, although silent renal artery stenosis may be present in many patients with vascular disease. Despite improvements in diagnostic and interventional techniques, controversy remains over whether, when, and how to revascularise the kidneys of patients with renal artery stenosis.

Pathophysiology

The pathophysiology of unilateral renal artery stenosis provides a clear example of how hypertension develops. Narrowing of the renal artery, due to atherosclerosis or, rarely, fibromuscular dysplasia, leads to reduced renal perfusion. The consequent activation of the renin-angiotensin system causes hypertension (mediated by angiotensin II), hypokalaemia, and hyponatraemia (which are features of secondary hyperaldosteronism). Although these features may be reversed by correcting the stenosis, a classic presentation is uncommon, and hypertension is rarely cured in patients with atheromatous renal artery stenosis. In addition, it is now known that renal artery stenosis is underdiagnosed and may present as a spectrum of disease from secondary hypertension to end stage renal failure, reflecting variation in the underlying disease process. Thus, the presence of overt, or coincidental, renal artery stenosis usually reflects widespread vascular disease, with the associated implications for cardiovascular risk and patient survival.

Clinical features

Atheromatous renal artery stenosis typically occurs in male smokers aged over 50 years with coexistent vascular disease elsewhere. It is underdiagnosed and may present with a spectrum of clinical manifestations. Although conventionally thought of as a cause of hypertension, atheromatous renal artery stenosis is not commonly associated with mild to moderate hypertension. However, it is present in up to a third of patients with malignant or drug resistant hypertension. Renal artery stenosis is a cause of end stage renal failure, and patients commonly present with chronic renal failure (with or without hypertension). Typical patients have a bland urine sediment and non-nephrotic range proteinuria, although occasional patients may have heavy proteinuria with focal glomerulosclerosis on renal biopsy. Patients may also present with acute renal failure, particularly those with bilateral renal artery stenosis (or stenosis of a single functioning kidney) who are taking drugs that block the renin-angiotensin system.

Less common presentations include recurrent, rapid onset ("flash") pulmonary oedema, which is probably a consequence of fluid retention, and diastolic ventricular dysfunction, which often accompanies (bilateral) atheromatous renal artery stenosis. Biochemical abnormalities may also be present in patients with modest or no serious renal impairment. Patients with unilateral renal artery stenosis have raised circulating concentrations of renin and aldosterone and associated hypokalaemia; in contrast to patients with primary hyperaldosteronism, their plasma sodium concentration is

---

Characteristics of renal artery stenosis

Fibromuscular dysplasia
- Young age group
- Predominantly affects women
- Presents as hypertension
- Rarely causes renal impairment

Atherosclerosis
- Older age group
- More common in men
- Affects smokers
- Evidence of atherosclerosis elsewhere
- Causes hypertension—often treatment resistant
- Often associated with renal impairment

Prevalence of atheromatous renal artery stenosis

- 27% of necropsies
- 25% of patients having routine coronary angiography
- 50% of patients having peripheral angiography
- 16-20% of all patients starting renal dialysis
- 25-30% of patients aged over 60 years on dialysis programmes

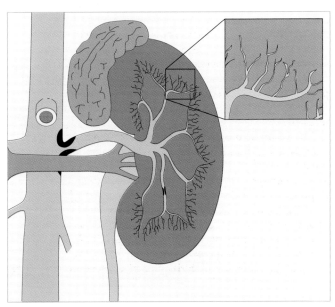

Atheromatous lesions may affect different sized vessels within the kidney, and multiple lesions may exist. The site limits the potential for revascularisation; only lesions within the large vessels are amenable. The commonest site, at the ostium of the renal artery, is more effectively treated by stenting. Ulcerated atheromatous plaques may also generate cholesterol microemboli (particularly after vascular intervention)

Clinical features and pointers to diagnosis of renal artery disease

- Young hypertensive patients with no family history (fibromuscular dysplasia)
- Peripheral vascular disease
- Resistant hypertension
- Deteriorating blood pressure control in compliant, long standing hypertensive patients
- Deterioration in renal function with angiotensin converting enzyme inhibition
- Renal impairment with minimal proteinuria
- "Flash" pulmonary oedema
- >1.5 cm difference in kidney size on ultrasonography
- Secondary hyperaldosteronism (low plasma sodium and potassium concentrations)

normal or reduced. Patients with bilateral renal artery stenosis commonly have impaired renal function.

Clinical examination often shows bruits over major vessels, including the abdominal aorta (a feature of widespread atherosclerosis), although the classic finding of lateralising bruits over the renal arteries is uncommon.

Diagnosis

The main differential diagnoses of atheromatous renal artery stenosis in patients with hypertension and renal impairment are benign hypertensive nephrosclerosis and cholesterol microembolic disease. Differentiating between these conditions may be difficult, particularly as all three can occur simultaneously.

Angiography remains the standard test for diagnosing atheromatous renal artery stenosis and is widely available. However, it is not without risk and may worsen renal function. Non-invasive imaging techniques are beginning to replace conventional angiography. Although acceptable results have been reported by single enthusiastic centres, it remains to be seen whether these can be reproduced. Each has its own limitation. Doppler ultrasonography is very operator sensitive and is often impossible in obese patients. Spiral computed tomography requires the use of iodinated contrast media and radiation. Isotope renography (with or without captopril) has the advantage of providing information on renal function but is of little value in bilateral disease or when renal function is seriously impaired. Magnetic resonance angiography is the most promising imaging technique. It requires no contrast and permits reconstruction of the image in different planes. However, use of this technique is limited by lack of access to magnetic resonance imaging machines in the United Kingdom.

All the above non-invasive tests require variable degrees of patient cooperation, particularly the ability to hold a breath for up to 30 seconds for image acquisition. Moreover, none of the available imaging techniques identify the patients who will respond to revascularisation. The aim of investigation is to establish the diagnosis and whether revascularisation is possible or appropriate. In practice we use ultrasonography to define renal size and symmetry before proceeding to angiography to delineate the lesion. Magnetic resonance angiography is reserved for patients at high risk of angiographic complications.

Prognosis

The rate of progression of atheromatous renal artery stenosis is difficult to evaluate accurately, and reports from large tertiary referral centres are likely to be biased by case mix as the studies have followed selected cohorts. Moreover, follow up may be limited by the influence of concomitant vascular disease on survival. Most studies (over a variable follow up period) estimate the risk of radiological progression of atheromatous renal artery stenosis to be about 50%, and risk is dependent on initial severity of the lesion. The rate of occlusion of renal arteries with greater than 60% stenosis is about 5% a year.

Patients who have bilateral atheromatous renal artery stenosis with an occluded renal artery are three times more likely to reach end stage renal failure within two years than patients who have bilateral disease without occlusion (50% v 18%). The rate of loss of functional renal tissue (implied by loss of renal size of ≥1 cm at one year after diagnosis) is about three times higher for patients with bilateral disease than for those with unilateral disease (43% v 13%).

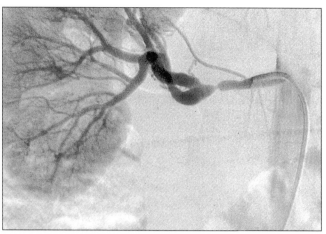

Angiogram of renal artery stenosis due to fibromuscular dysplasia of renal artery. Lesions typically affect the main renal artery, are beaded in appearance, and may have multiple stenoses

---

Non-invasive imaging techniques

- Doppler ultrasonography
- Captopril renography
- Spiral computed tomography
- Magnetic resonance angiography

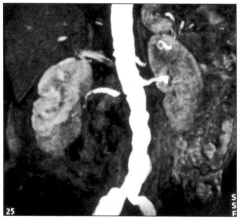

Gadolinium enhanced magnetic resonance angiogram showing a tight stenosis at the origin of the right renal artery. The left renal artery is normal

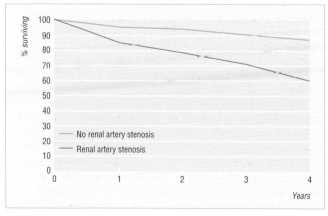

Effect of coexistent renal artery stenosis on survival among patients having coronary angiography

ABC of Arterial and Venous Disease

Treatment

Treatment of atheromatous renal artery stenosis must be tailored to the individual and should be undertaken in the expectation that revascularisation will prolong life. Hypertension in patients with renal artery stenosis can be controlled by drugs alone in almost 90% of cases. Angiotensin converting enzyme inhibitors reduce the glomerular filtration rate in about one third of patients with high grade bilateral atheromatous renal artery stenosis. Although this reduction is reversible in most cases, these drugs should be used with utmost caution.

Angioplasty is the traditional revascularisation procedure. Technical advances have revolutionised angioplasty, but few trials have examined its effects in renal artery stenosis. The available randomised controlled trials comparing drug treatment with angioplasty have shown only a modest reduction in blood pressure or antihypertensive drug requirements after angioplasty. Unlike treatment of fibromuscular dysplasia, cure of atheromatous renal artery stenosis by angioplasty alone is rare.

Treatment options for renal artery stenosis

- Drug treatment to reduce blood pressure (avoiding angiotensin converting enzyme inhibitors if possible)
- Stop smoking
- Lipid lowering treatment
- Preventive treatment for coexistent vascular disease, eg aspirin
- Angioplasty for non-ostial disease and fibromuscular dysplasia
- Stent insertion for ostial atheromatous renal artery stenosis
- Surgical bypass for failed endovascular procedures

Indications for revascularisation

- Resistant hypertension
- Deteriorating renal function
- Critical stenosis, or stenosis with deteriorating function, in single functioning kidney
- Fibromuscular dysplasia
- Associated heart failure ("flash" pulmonary oedema)

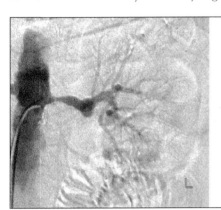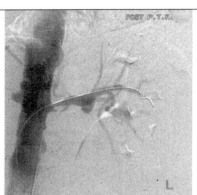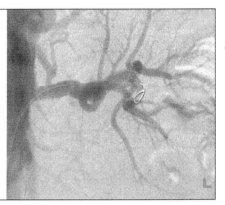

Endovascular treatment. In this ostial lesion (left) there is no improvement after angioplasty because of elastic recoil (middle). An excellent morphological result is then achieved by stent placement (right)

Most atheromatous renal artery stenosis is due to aortic plaques encroaching on the ostium of the renal artery. Angioplasty is less than ideal in this situation because of the elastic recoil of the aortic plaques. The introduction of stents has helped overcome this problem. A recent randomised controlled trial comparing stent insertion to angioplasty alone in patients with ostial stenosis found a higher initial success rate (88% v 57%) and lower restenosis rate at six months (14% v 48%) in patients who had a stent inserted. Apart from expense there is little to argue against a policy of primary stenting for ostial renal artery stenosis. Although the patency rates from surgical bypass are excellent, surgery should probably be reserved for patients in whom stenting fails or who develop complications.

Complications of intervention

- Groin haematoma
- Femoral artery false aneurysm
- Ischaemia distal to puncture site
- Contrast nephrotoxicity
- Renal artery occlusion, dissection, or perforation
- Cholesterol embolism syndrome

Benefits of revascularisation

Renal function may improve greatly after vascular intervention, although it is difficult to identify which patients will benefit and the potential of the kidney distal to the stenosis to recover function. The available studies in patients with mild to moderate renal impairment show that renal function improves in 25% of patients, remains stable in 50%, and deteriorates in 25% after surgical revascularisation or stenting. Renal length ≥8 cm on ultrasonography and the presence of intact glomeruli on renal biopsy have been suggested as good prognostic markers but have not been formally studied. Patients in whom renal function deteriorates after vascular intervention have an extremely poor prognosis, with most requiring dialysis or dying within one year.

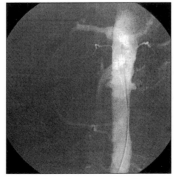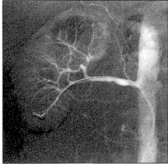

Occluded renal artery before (left) and after (right) successful stenting. It is possible to revascularise an occluded renal artery provided there is distal reconstitution of the renal artery with collateral vessels maintaining viability. In this relatively unusual case, the patient required dialysis at presentation but became dialysis independent after stenting

28

Although a modest improvement in blood pressure or a reduction in antihypertensive drug requirement may be the goal of revascularisation, renal protection may emerge as a more important factor. Animal studies have shown that renal tissue distal to renal artery stenosis undergoes irreversible ischaemic change, tubular atrophy, interstitial fibrosis, and glomerulosclerosis despite antihypertensive treatment. Although similar evidence is not available in humans, insertion of a stent in patients with renal artery stenosis slowed the rate of loss of renal function despite modest blood pressure benefits. A final reason to pursue revascularisation is the fact that patients with atheromatous renal artery stenosis have a worse prognosis than any other group on dialysis, with a median survival of 27 months, and prevention of progression to end stage renal failure may have greatest benefits in this group. The benefits of revascularisation, and the potential benefits of early intervention (for example, in patients with coincidental findings of renal artery stenosis) will need to be established by randomised controlled trials before the burden of additional procedures is placed on both radiologists and patients.

Special cases

Fibromuscular dysplasia is a much less common cause of renal artery stenosis. It principally occurs in young women, who present with unilateral disease, hypertension, and biochemical abnormalities. The lesions are graded by their distribution. In contrast to atheromatous renal artery stenosis, fibromuscular dysplasia is often cured by intervention, and often by angioplasty alone.

Patients with renal transplants have accelerated cardiovascular disease, one of the manifestations of which is the development of stenosis in the transplanted renal artery. This produces hypertension, fluid retention, and renal impairment similar to that found in patients with bilateral renal artery stenosis and is an indication for revascularisation.

Treatment recommendations

Recommending treatment for renal artery stenosis is difficult with the quality of the evidence available and the paucity of controlled trials. Surgical revascularisation is rarely indicated but may have a role in patients for whom angioplasty or stenting is not technically feasible or in patients with complex disease having abdominal vascular surgery. Nephrectomy (by minimally invasive surgery) may be considered in patients with unilateral disease whose blood pressure cannot be controlled because of a small or poorly functioning kidney.

Whatever recommendations we suggest, there will be disagreement. Firmly held, preconceived beliefs exist on the treatment of renal artery stenosis despite the fact that there have been few large outcome studies comparing treatment strategies. The ASTRAL (angioplasty and stent for renal artery lesions) study is a British randomised controlled trial that will compare angioplasty with and without stenting against drug treatment in 1000 patients with renal artery stenosis. Our future approach to the management of renal artery stenosis will depend on the conduct of relevant controlled trials.

The picture of gadolinium enhanced magnetic resonance angiography was provided by D Wilcock, Leicester Royal Infirmary.

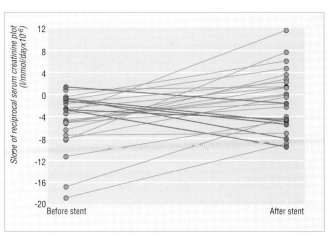

Effect of stent placement on rate of loss of renal function (expressed as slope of serum creatinine concentration with time). Overall, a significant reduction occurred in the rate of loss of renal function, although the individual response was variable

Further reading

- Mailloux LU, Napolitano B, Bellucci AG, Vernance M, Wilkes BM, Mossey RT. Renal vascular disease causing end-stage renal disease: incidence, clinical correlates and outcomes: a 20-year clinical experience. *Am J Kidney Dis* 1994;24:622-9.
- Plouin PF, Chatellier G, Darne B, Raynaud A. Blood pressure outcome of angioplasty in atherosclerotic renal artery stenosis: a randomized trial. Essai Multicentrique Medicaments vs Angioplastie (EMMA) Study Group. *Hypertension* 1998;31:823-9.
- Van de Ven PJG, Kaatee R, Beutler JJ, Beek FJ, Woittiez AJ, Buskens E et al. Arterial stenting and balloon angioplasty in ostial atherosclerotic renovascular disease: a randomised trial. *Lancet* 1999;353:282-6.
- Textor SC. Revascularisation in atherosclerotic renal artery disease. *Kidney Int* 1998;53:799-811.
- Conlon PJ, Athirakul K, Kovalik E, Schwab SJ, Crowley J, Stack R, et al. Survival in renovascular disease. *J Am Soc Nephrol* 1998;9:252-6.

Recommendations for treatment

Patient characteristics	Treatment
Controlled blood pressure Minimal renal impairment (creatinine <150 mmol/l) Renal artery stenosis <50% (unilateral or bilateral)	Medical
Advanced renal failure and Renal size <8 cm or Renal artery occlusion (without distal recanalisation) or No evidence of renal function in affected kidney or Biopsy showing severe irreversible changes	No prospect of recovery with intervention
Renal size >8 cm and renal artery stenosis >50% and Poorly controlled blood pressure or Deterioration in renal function with angiotensin converting enzyme inhibitors or Progressive renal impairment	Angioplasty for non-ostial lesions Angioplasty plus stent for ostial disease

8 Arterial aneurysms

M M Thompson, P R F Bell

True arterial aneurysms are defined as a 50% increase in the normal diameter of the vessel. Clinical symptoms usually arise from the common complications that affect arterial aneurysms—namely, rupture, thrombosis, or distal embolisation. Although the aneurysmal process may affect any large or medium sized artery, the most commonly affected vessels are the aorta and iliac arteries, followed by the popliteal, femoral, and carotid vessels.

Abdominal aortic aneurysms

Aneurysms of the infrarenal abdominal aorta and iliac arteries coexist to such a degree that they may be considered a single clinical entity. Abdominal aneurysms usually affect elderly men (>65 years), with a prevalence of 5%. In England, abdominal aneurysm is responsible for over 11 000 hospital admissions and 10 000 deaths a year. Interestingly, unlike other atherosclerotic vascular disorders, the prevalence of abdominal aortic aneurysms is increasing rapidly, and aneurysmal rupture is now the 13th commonest cause of death in the Western world.

Clinical presentation
Although abdominal aneurysms may cause symptoms because of pressure on surrounding structures, about three quarters remain asymptomatic at initial diagnosis. With the exception of vague abdominal pain, clinical symptoms usually result from embolisation or rupture of the aneurysm.

The appearance of microembolic lower limb infarcts in a patient with easily palpable pedal pulses may suggest the presence of either popliteal or abdominal aneurysms. Additionally, patients with embolisation of mural thrombus from an abdominal aneurysm may present with acute limb ischaemia due to femoral or popliteal occlusion.

The diagnostic triad of hypovolaemic shock, pulsatile abdominal mass, and abdominal or back pain is encountered in only a minority of patients with ruptured abdominal aneurysms. In general, ruptured abdominal aortic aneurysm should be considered in any patient with hypotension and atypical abdominal symptoms. Similarly, the presence of abdominal pain in a patient with a known aneurysm or pulsatile mass must be considered to represent a rapidly expanding or ruptured aneurysm and be treated accordingly. In the community setting, the death rate from ruptured abdominal aortic aneurysms is almost 90%, as 80% of patients will die before reaching hospital and about 50% die during surgery to repair the rupture.

Methods of diagnosis
The sensitivity of abdominal palpation to detect aortic aneurysms increases with the diameter of the aneurysm, but palpation is not sufficiently reliable for routine diagnosis. Similarly, plain abdominal radiography shows a calcified aneurysmal aortic wall in only half of cases.

The simplest diagnostic test is B mode ultrasonography, which gives an accurate assessment of both the diameter and the site of the aneurysm. If more accurate morphological data are required to determine the exact relation of the aneurysm to the visceral or renal arteries, detailed cross sectional imaging may be obtained by computed tomography or magnetic resonance angiography.

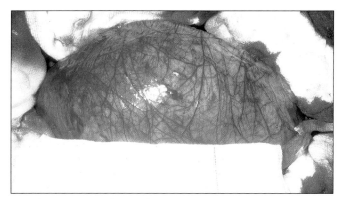

Large infrarenal abdominal aortic aneurysm before surgical repair

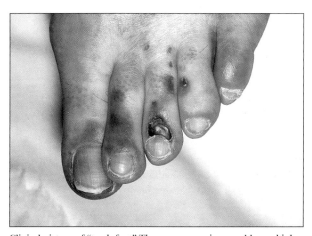

Clinical picture of "trash foot." The appearance is caused by multiple microscopic atheromatous emboli from a large infrarenal aortic aneurysm. The presence of digital infarcts in a patient with easily palpable pulses may point to an aneurysmal source of emboli

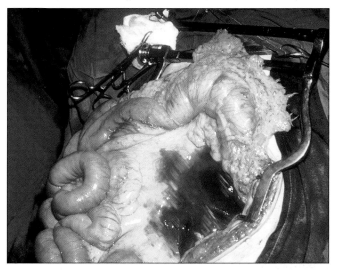

Ruptured abdominal aneurysm. Rupture usually occurs posteriorly into the retroperitoneum, which produces a contained leak and allows the possibility of surgical repair. Free anterior intraperitoneal rupture usually results in exsanguination

The diagnosis of ruptured abdominal aortic aneurysms relies on clinical symptoms. Ultrasonography is used to confirm an aneurysm if it is difficult to palpate. Computed tomography has a low specificity (about 75%) for determining the presence of a rupture and adds little information to routine clinical assessment.

Indications for surgery

Elective surgery

The decision to operate on a patient with an asymptomatic abdominal aneurysm is based on an analysis of the risk of aneurysmal rupture compared with the mortality of elective surgical repair. The risk of rupture is related to many factors, but the diameter of the aortic aneurysm has historically been used as the principal determinant.

Unfortunately, little information is available on the rupture rates of large abdominal aneurysms, but pooled analysis of existing data suggests that the risk of rupture increases exponentially in aneurysms above 55-60 mm. This has led to a broad surgical consensus that aneurysms exceeding 55 mm in diameter should be surgically repaired if there are no confounding factors that would substantially increase the risk of elective surgery.

The treatment for smaller aneurysms has recently been clarified by the UK small aneurysm trial, which studied 1090 patients with aneurysms of 40-55 mm. The study found a 30 day operative mortality of 5.8%, mean risk of rupture for small aneurysms of 1% a year, and no difference in survival between treatment groups at two, four, or six years. The cost for early surgery was higher than for surveillance, but early surgery was associated with improvement in some measures of quality of life.

Emergency treatment

Patients with suspected ruptured aneurysms should be considered for emergency surgical repair. Several studies have looked at preoperative risk factors and survival after emergency repair of an aneurysm. Although there is no precise scoring system that will allow accurate prediction of survival, the presence of several predictive factors (age > 80 years, unconsciousness, low haemoglobin concentration, cardiac arrest, severe cardiorespiratory disease) can be used to determine patients in whom the risk of dying during surgery approaches 100%.

Patients with symptomatic aneurysms should be treated as urgent cases and have the aneurysm repaired. The aetiology of pain from abdominal aneurysms is not well understood, although it has been attributed to stretching of the aneurysm sac or severe inflammation within the aneurysm wall (inflammatory aneurysms, see below).

Conventional surgical repair

Traditional surgical repair for asymptomatic abdominal aortic aneurysms involves exposure of the abdominal aorta, aortic and iliac clamping, and replacement of the aneurysmal segment with a prosthetic graft. Graft replacement is an effective, durable procedure, and most centres report 30 day mortality of about 5%, although this varies with the volume of work and type of hospital.

The mortality associated with surgical repair of aneurysms is closely related to the "fitness" of the patient for surgery; patients with severe cardiorespiratory disease have a perioperative mortality approaching 40%, with most deaths caused by cardiac events.

Endovascular repair

One of the major developments in vascular surgery over the past five years has been the introduction of endovascular repair of aneurysms. This technique uses an endoprosthesis, which is

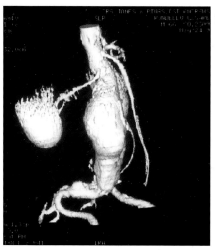

Computed tomogram showing large infrarenal abdominal aortic aneurysm

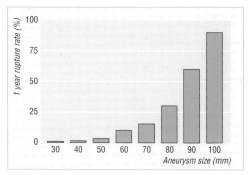

Annual rupture rates of abdominal aortic aneurysms according to size (based on pooled available data)

Factors predisposing to rupture of abdominal aortic aneurysms

- Diameter of aneurysm
- Diastolic blood pressure
- Chronic obstructive pulmonary disease
- Smoking
- Family history of ruptured aneurysm
- Expansion rate
- Intrinsic biology—inflammation within the aortic wall
- Thrombus-free surface area of aneurysm sac

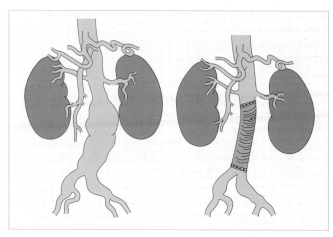

Conventional repair of abdominal aortic aneurysm. The aneurysmal segment of the aortoiliac segment is replaced with a prosthetic vascular graft (usually Dacron or ePTFE), which is sutured to the normal arterial "cuffs" above and below the aneurysm

delivered through the femoral arteries, to exclude an aneurysm from the circulation. The endograft is secured to the normal calibre aorta and iliac arteries using metallic expandable stents and relies on subsequent thrombosis of the aneurysm to abolish the risk of rupture.

Endovascular repair has several theoretical advantages over conventional surgery, and early evidence suggests that endovascular surgery is better for patients with coexistent disease, who would be high risk for conventional surgery. However, the long term durability of endovascular techniques is unknown, although experience so far shows that up to a quarter of patients undergoing endovascular aneurysm repair will require subsequent endovascular interventions to ensure regression of the aneurysm sac. A multicentre trial of endovascular repair and conventional surgery has started in the United Kingdom.

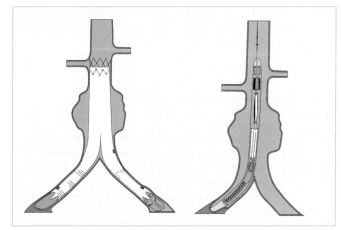

Endovascular aneurysm repair. The aneurysm sac is excluded by an endograft, which is introduced through a remote arteriotomy and anchored above and below the aneurysm sac

Potential advantages of endovascular repair over conventional surgery

- No need for abdominal incision
- Avoidance of aortic cross clamping
- No retroperitoneal dissection
- Improved perioperative cardiorespiratory function
- Reduction in metabolic stress response to aortic aneurysm repair
- Improved renal and gastrointestinal function
- Reduced hospital stay

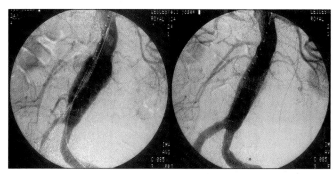

Aortoiliac aneurysm before and after exclusion by a bifurcated endovascular graft

Screening and medical treatment

Ultrasonography-based screening programmes to detect and treat asymptomatic aneurysms have been proposed as a mechanism to reduce the mortality from ruptured abdominal aortic aneurysms. Screening studies report a 2.5% prevalence of abdominal aortic aneurysms larger than 40 mm in men aged over 60 years.

Advocates of community screening have suggested that a single abdominal scan in men aged 65 would exclude 90% of the population from future aneurysm rupture, and long term follow up of screened and control populations in Chichester showed an 85% reduction in rupture in the screened group. A multicentre randomised trial is currently investigating the cost-effectiveness of community based aneurysm screening.

One of the problems with screening programmes is that it identifies many people with small aneurysms. These patients are not offered any form of treatment other than ultrasonographic surveillance, which may have implications for quality of life. However, recent studies have begun to elucidate the molecular and biochemical mechanisms of aneurysm formation, and clinical trials of the effectiveness of several groups of drugs to reduce expansion of small aneurysms are likely. The most promising of these drugs in experimental studies have been inhibitors of matrix metalloproteinases.

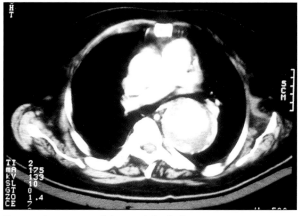

Inflammatory abdominal aneurysm. The aneurysm is typically white in appearance and densely adherent to surrounding structures. The duodenum is being mobilised from the aneurysm sac by sharp dissection

Variants of abdominal aneurysms

Inflammatory aneurysms

Inflammatory aneurysms are characterised by a dense inflammatory infiltrate within the aneurysm wall. They are typically white in appearance and may be densely adherent to surrounding structures, which could account for the increased operative mortality in affected patients Patients typically present with fever, malaise, and abdominal pain.

Thoracoabdominal aneurysms

Thoracoabdominal aneurysms extend to a variable degree from the thoracic aorta into the abdominal aorta. They

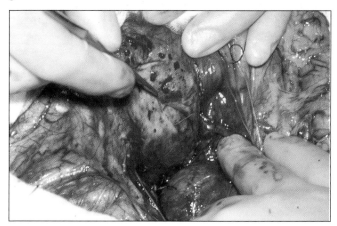

Computed tomogram of thoracoabdominal aneurysm

typically affect the origins of the visceral and renal arteries, which must be reimplanted into the graft during repair of the aneurysm. Mortality from repair of thoracoabdominal aneurysms is significantly higher than that for infrarenal surgery.

Peripheral aneurysms

Popliteal aneurysms comprise 80% of all peripheral aneurysms and usually exceed 20 mm in diameter. They are associated with aortic aneurysms (40% of cases), and are frequently bilateral (50%). In contrast to abdominal aortic aneurysms, patients with popliteal aneurysms usually present with acute limb ischaemia secondary to aneurysm thrombosis or distal embolisation. A diagnosis of popliteal aneurysms is suggested by easily palpable popliteal pulses and confirmed by duplex ultrasonography.

Patients who develop acute limb ischaemia due to popliteal thrombosis or embolism have a relatively poor prognosis (15% amputation rate) because of occlusion of the run off vessels. In these cases patients should have saphenous vein bypass and ligation of the popliteal aneurysm with clearance of the crural vessels by balloon thrombectomy or thrombolysis. The indications for elective surgery for asymptomatic popliteal aneurysms are based on suggestive evidence only, with most clinicians opting for surgical treatment when the aneurysm exceeds 25 mm in diameter. Results of bypass of asymptomatic popliteal aneurysms are excellent, with five year graft patency of 80% and limb salvage of 98%.

Femoral artery aneurysms are the second commonest peripheral aneurysm. Patients present with local pressure symptoms, thrombosis, or distal embolisation. Surgical treatment of true femoral aneurysms relies on the principles of excluding the aneurysm and restoration of blood flow in the limb.

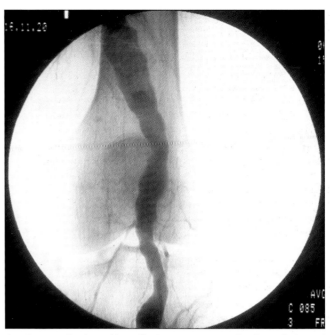

Arteriogram of patient with popliteal artery aneurysm showing typical spiralling appearance of the superficial femoral and popliteal arteries

Key references

- Thompson MM, Sayers RD. Arterial aneurysms. In: Beard JD, Gaines P, eds. *Companion to specialist surgical practice. Vol VII. Arterial surgery*. London: W B Saunders, 1998.
- UK Small Aneurysm Trial Participants. Mortality results for randomised controlled trial of early elective surgery or ultrasonographic surveillance for small abdominal aortic aneurysms. *Lancet* 1998;352:1649-55.
- Scott RAP, Wilson NM, Ashton HA, Kay DM. Influence of screening on the incidence of ruptured abdominal aortic aneurysm: 5-year results of a randomised controlled study. *Br J Surg* 1995;82:1066-70.

9 Secondary prevention of peripheral vascular disease

Sean Tierney, Fiona Fennessy, David Bouchier Hayes

Most patients with peripheral vascular disease may be reassured that, with respect to their legs, the condition usually runs a benign course. Less than one third of patients will require any surgical or radiological intervention and only 5% will have amputation. However, peripheral vascular disease is an independent predictor of increased risk of cardiovascular death. Half of patients presenting with peripheral vascular disease have symptoms of coronary artery disease or electrocardiographic abnormality, 90% have abnormalities on coronary angiography, and 40% have duplex evidence of carotid artery disease.

Symptomatic peripheral vascular disease carries at least a 30% risk of death within five years and almost 50% within 10 years, primarily due to myocardial infarction (60%) or stroke (12%). The risks are more than doubled in patients with severe disease (requiring surgery), but even asymptomatic patients (ankle brachial pressure index < 0.9) have a twofold to fivefold increased risk of fatal or non-fatal cardiovascular events.

Although modification of risk factors has not been shown to prevent progression of peripheral vascular disease or loss of limbs, detection of disease mandates an aggressive approach to modifying risk factors in order to reduce the risk of fatal and non-fatal myocardial infarction and stroke. The approach to risk reduction in patients with peripheral vascular disease is based on extrapolation from results of large studies of patients with coronary artery disease.

Modification of risk factors

Effective reduction of the risk of cardiovascular disease depends on coordinated and stringent modification of identifiable risk factors to prevent progression or new disease and the use of drugs to correct existing abnormalities. Stopping smoking, correction of hyperlipidaemia and hypertension, and optimisation of diabetic control are the cornerstones of secondary prevention of cardiovascular disease. Lesser benefits are also likely to accrue through weight reduction in obese patients, the institution of regular exercise, and dietary modification. Additional risk factors have been identified but are uncommon and their treatment is of unproved value.

Cigarette smoking

Cigarette smoking contributes to a third of all deaths from coronary artery disease, doubles the risk of stroke, and is almost ubiquitous among patients with peripheral vascular disease. Synergy between smoking and other risk factors substantially increases the risks of cardiovascular death associated with these factors. After a myocardial infarction or stroke, the risk of recurrence is reduced by 50% in those who stop smoking (even among long term heavy smokers). Firm evidence also exists that stopping smoking increases walking distance by twofold to threefold in 85% of patients with intermittent claudication. Furthermore, in patients requiring surgical bypass, patency rates are better among those who successfully stop smoking.

Because as few as 4% of established smokers in the general population successfully stop smoking without assistance, measures to improve on this are essential in the secondary prevention of cardiovascular disease. Modern smokers are clearly able to ignore punitive taxes and health warnings on

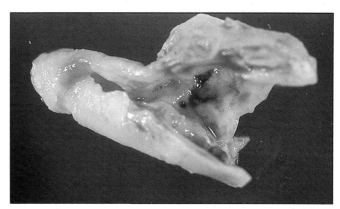

Excised atherosclerotic plaque

All patients with peripheral vascular disease should have their risk factors for coronary artery disease assessed and, if appropriate, modified according to current guidelines

---

Risk factors for cardiovascular disease

- Cigarette smoking
- Hyperlipidaemia
- Hypertension
- Diabetes mellitus
- Obesity
- Physical inactivity
- Diet high in saturated fats
- Hyperhomocysteinaemia
- Raised Lp(a) lipoprotein concentrations
- Hypercoagulable states

Study	Experimental	Control	Peto odds ratio	Peto odds ratio (95% CI)
Gum (46 studies) $\chi^2 = 54.5$	1405/7235	1065/9247		1.63 (1.48 to 1.78)
Patch (30 studies) $\chi^2 = 34.33$	1225/8929	458/7903		1.77 (1.58 to 1.97)
Intranasal spray (46 studies) $\chi^2 = 1.22$	107/448	52/439		2.27 (1.61 to 3.20)
Inhaler (4 studies) $\chi^2 = 1.34$	84/490	44/486		2.08 (1.43 to 3.04)
Sublingual (2 studies) $\chi^2 = 0.1$	49/243	31/245		1.73 (1.07 to 2.80)

0.1 0.2   1   5 10

Favours control   Favours treatment

Summary of results of meta-analysis of nicotine gum, patch, intranasal spray, and sublingual tablet versus control for stopping smoking. Maximum follow up 6-12 months

packaging. They respond better to short (5-10 minutes) counselling from doctors, particularly if they are recovering from myocardial infarction (50% success rates). Rates of stopping smoking have been increased to 70% by the addition of telephone based counselling.

Surprisingly, only half of current smokers in one study had been encouraged to stop smoking, and fewer had been specifically counselled. Hospitals caring for patients with cardiovascular disease can help by offering support programmes. The use of nicotine replacement (chewing gum or patches), which is safe for patients with stable cardiovascular disease, is effective when combined with counselling.

Measures to encourage stopping smoking

- Public health education
- Taxes
- Smoke free hospitals and workplace
- Advice from doctor
- Nurse case managers
- Support groups and counselling
- Nicotine replacement therapy

Hyperlipidaemia

Epidemiological data clearly indicate an association between total cholesterol concentration and the risk of cardiovascular death. Dietary measures may reduce serum cholesterol and low density lipoprotein cholesterol concentrations by about 10%, but long term compliance is poor.

The use of statins (hydroxymethylglutaryl coenzyme A reductase inhibitors) to lower total and low density lipoprotein cholesterol concentrations by 30-40% reduces the risk of cardiovascular death by up to 42% among patients younger than 70 years with established disease. The only statins licensed for secondary prevention are simvastatin and pravastatin. Statins also reduce triglyceride concentrations. Patients with severe dyslipidaemia require specialised treatment.

Although there are no published studies examining the effect of lipid reduction in patients with isolated peripheral vascular disease, patients with peripheral disease are included as a subgroup in current large trials such as the heart protection study and the Medical Research Council bezafibrate in patients with lower extremity arterial disease (LEADER) trial study. Because of their high risk of ischaemic heart disease patients with peripheral vascular disease who have a serum cholesterol concentration over 5.5 mmol/l should be treated. All patients should therefore have their lipid concentrations measured even if they do not require specific treatment for their peripheral vascular disease.

Dietary modifications in hyperlipidaemia

- Reduce total fat intake (<30% of total energy)
- Reduce saturated fat intake (<7% of energy) and substitute with unsaturates
- Decrease dietary cholesterol intake (<200 mg/day)
- Increase fibre intake
- Moderate alcohol intake
- Aim for ideal body mass index (21-25)

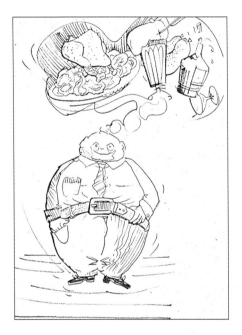

Diabetes mellitus

The adverse effect of diabetes on serum lipid concentrations and the accelerated atheromatous process in diabetic patients act synergistically with the result that 80% die of cardiovascular disease. The atheromatous process particularly affects smaller more distal vessels, which makes surgical reconstruction more difficult or impossible. Diabetic patients are therefore more likely to require amputation than other patients with peripheral vascular disease. Modification of other risk factors is particularly important in this population, and the absolute benefits of reducing cholesterol concentration are likely to be greater in diabetic patients.

Poor glycaemic control in patients with type 2 diabetes is associated with an increased risk of cardiovascular complications, but the value of tighter control in preventing major cardiac events remains unclear. However, tight glycaemic control has beneficial effects on serum lipid concentrations, and the DIGAMI (diabetes insulin glucose after myocardial infarction) study showed that improved glycaemic control benefits patients after myocardial infarction. Careful attention to foot care is particularly important in diabetic patients with peripheral vascular disease.

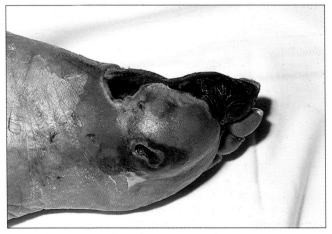

Foot of diabetic patient with peripheral vascular disease

Hypertension

The rationale for treating hypertension is largely based on its adverse effects on the heart and cerebrovascular system. Conventional guidelines such as those produced by the second working party of the British Hypertension Society are applicable to patients with peripheral vascular disease. Although it might seem preferable to use vasodilators in patients with peripheral vascular disease, β blockers are safe if they are required to obtain adequate blood pressure control.

Specific therapeutic measures

Diet
Observational studies suggest that diets rich in fish, fruit, vegetables, and fibre but low in saturated fat may protect against cardiovascular disease. Dietary supplementation with fish oil (which is rich in n-3 polyunsaturated fatty acids) has recently been shown to protect against cardiovascular death after myocardial infarction in a large trial, but other trials have failed to find such a benefit.

Vitamins and trace elements may also alter cardiovascular risk through other mechanisms. Antioxidants (vitamins E and C) help prevent the oxidation of low density lipoprotein cholesterol, which is a key step in the atherogenic process. Studies in patients with peripheral vascular disease have shown no specific benefits of antioxidants, but no large scale trials have been done.

Cardiovascular risk is independently related to plasma homocysteine concentrations, and it has been proposed that dietary supplementation with folic acid (which reduces homocysteine concentrations) may aid in the primary prevention of cardiovascular disease. However, no large prospective trials have been done. Severe hyperhomocysteinaemia (> 10 µmol/l), which may respond to vitamin supplementation, should be considered in patients with premature atherosclerotic disease without other risk factors. In the absence of strong evidence for routine vitamin supplementation, the most prudent approach is to recommend a balanced diet rich in fruit, vegetables, and whole grains.

Exercise
Physical rehabilitation programmes form an important part of reducing the risk of cardiovascular disease. If no supervised exercise programme is available, patients with intermittent claudication should be advised to walk for an hour a day, pausing to rest whenever claudication pain develops. This results in a 20-200% improvement in walking distance. Although it has been suggested that repeated ischaemia-reperfusion injury provoked by walking might have deleterious systemic effects, regular exercise actually reduces concentrations of serum inflammatory markers.

Antiplatelet therapy
Aspirin has been proved effective in the secondary prevention of cardiovascular events and death in patients with established atherosclerosis. Patients with peripheral vascular disease who do not have specific contraindications should receive 75 mg aspirin daily. The cost effectiveness of newer antiplatelet drugs remains to be determined.

Conclusion

Although individual specialties tend to treat arterial lesions in isolation, this approach ignores the real risk to patients from the

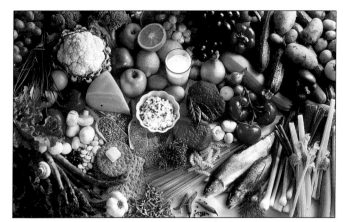
A balanced diet rich in fruit, vegetables, and fish may protect against cardiovascular disease

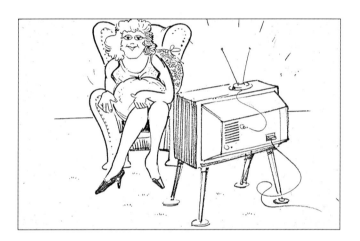

Further reading

- Bainton D, Sweetnam P, Baker I, Elwood P. Peripheral vascular disease: consequence for survival and association with risk factors in the Speedwell prospective heart disease study. *Br Heart J* 1994;72:128-32.
- Leng GC, Price JF, Jepson RG. Lipid-lowering for lower limb atherosclerosis. In: *Cochrane Library*. Issue 4. Oxford: Update Software, 1999.
- Scottish Intercollegiate Guidelines Network. Lipids and the primary prevention of coronary heart disease. *SIGN* 1999;40.
- Department of Health. *Standing medical advisory statement on the use of statins.* Leeds: DoH, 1997. (Circular EL (97) 41.)
- O'Brien E, Bouchier Hayes D, Fitzgerald D, Atkins N. The arterial organ in cardiovascular disease: ADAPT (arterial disease assessment, prevention, and treatment) clinic. *Lancet* 1998;352:1700-1.
- American Heart Association Writing Group. Optimal risk factor management in the patient after coronary revascularization. americanheart.org/Scientific/statements/1994/129401.html
- American Heart Association. Antioxidant consumption and risk of coronary heart disease: emphasis on vitamin C, vitamin E, and beta carotene. *Circulation* 1999; 99:591-5.

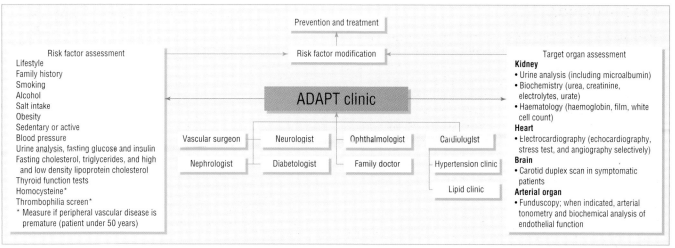

Arterial disease assessment, prevention, and treatment (ADAPT) clinics provide a common strategy for all patients with cardiovascular disease regardless of target organ affected

effects of the same disease on other vascular beds. Although simple measures (diet, exercise, stopping smoking) may be adequate for some, the management of many patients is complex. Patients at high risk of cardiovascular disease are best managed in an integrated fashion, and the concept of an arterial disease assessment, prevention, and treatment clinic to overcome the often haphazard management of risk factors seems the best way forward. Precise risk can be determined by using a computer program based on history, examination, and laboratory results and a specific programme of modification instituted and monitored. This holistic approach to the management of cardiovascular disease is the best way to minimise the risk of disease progression and premature death in patients with peripheral vascular disease.

The meta-analysis data on nicotine replacement therapy were taken from Silagy et al. *Cochrane library*. Issue 4. Oxford: Update Software, 1999.

The picture of fruit, vegetables and fish is reproduced with permission from Cephas Photo Library.

10 Vasculitis

C O S Savage, L Harper, P Cockwell, D Adu, A J Howie

Vasculitis is inflammation of blood vessel walls. The clinical and pathological features are variable and depend on the site and type of blood vessels that are affected. Diseases in which vasculitis is a primary process are called primary systemic vasculitides.

The main types of vasculitides can be described using clinical features and pathological findings according to the Chapel Hill Consensus Conference. These names and definitions will be followed in this article. Definitive classification of systemic vasculitis is unsatisfactory since aetiology and pathogenesis are rarely known, and clinical and histological features overlap. Vasculitis may also occur as a secondary feature in other diseases, such as systemic lupus erythematosus and rheumatoid arthritis.

Fever, night sweats, malaise, myalgia, and arthralgia are common in all types of vasculitis. Active vasculitis is usually associated with an acute phase response with an increase in C reactive protein concentration, erythrocyte sedimentation rate, or plasma viscosity.

Large vessel vasculitis

Giant cell arteritis (temporal arteritis)

Clinical features include unilateral throbbing headache, facial pain, and claudication of the jaw when eating. Visual loss is a feared symptom and may be sudden and painless, affecting part or all of the visual field. Diplopia may also occur. Giant cell arteritis is the most common type of primary systemic vasculitis with an incidence of 200/million population/year.

Treatment is with high dose corticosteroids (40-60 mg/day), which should be started as soon as the diagnosis is suspected to avoid visual loss. The diagnosis is confirmed by biopsy of the affected artery, done within 24 hours of starting corticosteroids. The corticosteroid dose may be reduced to 10 mg/day over six months and then more slowly to a maintenance of 5-10 mg/day. Maintenance treatment may be required for two years. The disease is monitored by measuring C reactive protein concentrations, erythrocyte sedimentation rate, or plasma viscosity.

Takayasu's arteritis

Takayasu's arteritis is most common in Asia and the Far East and affects women more than men. Disease of the arteries supplying the arms, head, neck, and heart leads to the aortic arch syndrome with claudication of the arm, loss of arm pulses, variation in blood pressure of more than 10 mm Hg between the arms, arterial bruits, angina, aortic regurgitation, syncope, stroke, and visual disturbance. The descending aortic syndrome may cause bowel ischaemia or infarction, renovascular hypertension, and renal impairment.

Diagnosis is by angiography or magnetic resonance angiography. Treatment of acute disease in patients with high C reactive protein concentration or erythrocyte sedimentation rate is with corticosteroids. Cytotoxic drugs such as cyclophosphamide can be added if steroids alone do not control the disease. Surgery or angioplasty may be required for stenoses once active inflammation has been controlled.

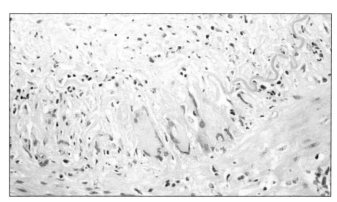
Temporal artery biopsy specimen with giant cell inflammation

Definitions of large vessel vasculitis

Giant cell arteritis (temporal arteritis)
- Granulomatous arteritis of aorta and its major branches, especially extracranial branches of carotid artery
- Often affects temporal artery
- Usually occurs in patients older than 50 years
- Often associated with polymyalgia rheumatica

Takayasu's arteritis
- Granulomatous inflammation of aorta and its major branches
- Usually occurs in patients younger than 50 years

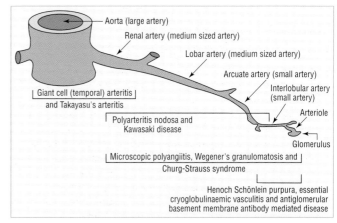
Spectrum of systemic vasculitides organised according to predominant size of vessels affected (adapted from Jennette et al, Arthritis Rheum 1994;37:187-92)

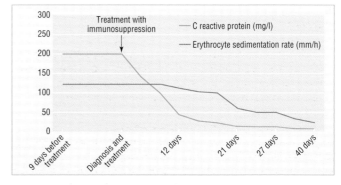
C reactive protein concentration (>10 mg/l) and erythrocyte sedimentation rate (>18 mm/h) are raised at time of diagnosis of giant cell arteritis but fall to normal levels after starting immunosuppressant therapy

Medium vessel vasculitis

Polyarteritis nodosa

Polyarteritis nodosa is uncommon in the United Kingdom. It is associated with hepatitis B virus in some patients. Arterial disease leads to ischaemia or infarction within affected organs. The condition can affect the gut causing bleeding or perforation, the heart causing angina or myocardial infarction, the kidneys causing cortical infarcts leading to hypertension and renal failure, and the peripheral nerves causing mononeuritis multiplex. Hepatitis may reflect the presence of hepatitis B virus.

Diagnosis is based on the presence of arterial aneurysms on angiography of the renal, hepatic, splanchnic, or splenic circulations. Biopsy of affected muscle or nerve may confirm the presence of vasculitis. Treatment of polyarteritis associated with hepatitis B virus requires an antiviral drug such as interferon alfa combined with short course, high dose corticosteroids and plasma exchange. Non-hepatitis B virus polyarteritis usually responds to corticosteroids alone, although cyclophosphamide may be required for patients with more severe disease.

Kawasaki disease

Kawasaki disease affects children, usually under the age of 12 years. In Japan the incidence exceeds 100/100 000 children younger than 5 years but is less than 5/100 000 in this age group in the United Kingdom.

The most serious feature of Kawasaki disease is coronary artery disease; aneurysms occur in a fifth of untreated patients and may lead to myocardial infarction. They can be detected by echocardiography. High dose intravenous immunoglobulins reduce the prevalence of coronary artery aneurysms, provided that treatment is started within 10 days of onset of the disease. Low dose aspirin is recommended for thrombocythaemia.

Small vessel vasculitis associated with antineutrophil cytoplasmic antibody

Small vessel vasculitides are being recognised more frequently, mainly because of increased awareness. Estimates of incidence have increased from fewer than 5 cases per million population in the early 1980s to over 20 per million. The early symptoms of these disorders are non-specific with fever, malaise, arthralgia, myalgia, and weight loss, and patients in whom such symptoms are persistent should be screened for antineutrophil cytoplasmic antibodies (ANCA); have their erythrocyte sedimentation rate and C reactive protein concentration measured; and have their urine tested for blood with a dipstick. Early diagnosis is essential to prevent potentially life threatening renal and pulmonary injury. Delays in diagnosis are unfortunately common, and this often leads to serious morbidity. Once respiratory or renal disease develops, the course is usually rapidly progressive.

Wegener's granulomatosis

Upper respiratory tract disease occurs in more than 90% of cases and includes sinusitis; nasal crusting, bleeding, obstruction, and collapse of the nasal bridge; serous otitis media with conductive deafness; and tracheal stenosis. Limited Wegener's refers to disease that affects only the respiratory tract at the time of diagnosis; many cases evolve to systemic disease. Lung disease is common with cough, haemoptysis, and dyspnoea and may progress to life threatening pulmonary haemorrhage. The kidneys are affected in up to 80% of cases; blood, protein, and casts are present in the urine and should be examined by dipstick testing and microscopy. If untreated, there is loss of renal function, often within days. Other features include purpuric rashes, nail fold infarcts, and ocular manifestations including

---

Definitions of medium sized vessel vasculitis

Polyarteritis nodosa
- Necrotising inflammation of medium and small arteries without glomerulonephritis, pulmonary capillaritis, or disease of other arterioles, capillaries, or venules

Kawasaki disease
- Arteritis affecting large, medium, and small arteries and associated with mucocutaneous lymph node syndrome
- Coronary arteries are usually affected and aorta and veins may be affected
- Usually occurs in children

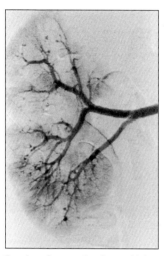

Renal angiogram showing multiple arterial aneurysms

Features of mucocutaneous lymph node syndrome in Kawasaki disease

- Fever for >5 days
- Conjunctival congestion
- Changes to lips and oral cavity: dry, red, fissured lips; strawberry tongue; reddening of oral and pharyngeal mucosa
- Changes of peripheral extremities: red palms and soles; indurative oedema; desquamation of finger tips during convalescence
- Macular polymorphous rash on trunk
- Swollen cervical lymph nodes

At least five features must be present

Definitions for diagnosis of vasculitides often associated with antineutrophil cytoplasm antibodies

Wegener's granulomatosis
- Granulomatous inflammation of the respiratory tract
- Necrotising vasculitis affecting small to medium sized vessels (capillaries, venules, arterioles, and arteries)
- Necrotising glomerulonephritis is common

Microscopic polyangiitis (microscopic polyarteritis)
- Necrotising vasculitis with few or no immune deposits affecting small vessels (capillaries, venules, arterioles, and arteries)
- Necrotising arteritis of small and medium sized arteries may be present
- Necrotising glomerulonephritis very common
- Pulmonary capillaritis often occurs

Churg-Strauss syndrome
- Eosinophil rich and granulomatous inflammation of respiratory tract
- Necrotising vasculitis affecting small to medium sized vessels
- Blood eosinophilia ($>1.5 \times 10^9/l$)
- Usually associated with asthma

conjunctival haemorrhages, scleritis, uveitis, keratitis, proptosis, or ocular muscle paralysis due to retro-orbital inflammation. The disease can affect the gut causing haemorrhage, the heart causing coronary artery ischaemia, and the neurological system causing sensory neuropathy or mononeuritis multiplex.

The two pathological hallmarks of Wegener's disease are chronic granulomatous inflammation and vasculitis. Granulomas (localised microscopic collections of macrophages) are not always present. Granulomas in the lung may coalesce into large masses which cavitate. The vasculitis affects capillaries particularly in the lung, causing lung haemorrhage, and glomeruli, causing glomerulonephritis that may be segmental, global, focal, or diffuse with thrombosis, necrosis of capillary loops, and accumulation of cells in Bowman's space. Affected arteries or arterioles show an inflammatory infiltrate and fibrinoid necrosis. There is no deposition of immunoglobulins within the kidney or vessel walls.

Microscopic polyangiitis (microscopic polyarteritis)

Microscopic polyangiitis has many similarities to Wegener's granulomatosis, but disease of the upper respiratory tract is uncommon in microscopic polyangiitis, although pulmonary haemorrhage may occur. Patients with microscopic polyangiitis usually have glomerulonephritis, and, rarely, disease may be limited to the kidney. No granuloma formation is seen.

Diagnosis

Diagnosis is based on typical clinical features, biopsy (usually of kidney, occasionally of nasal mucosa or lung) and presence of antineutrophil cytoplasmic antibodies. These antibodies usually have specificity for the enzymes proteinase-3 or myeloperoxidase and can be detected by enzyme linked immunosorbent assay (ELISA). In indirect immunofluorescence tests, antineutrophil cytoplasmic antibodies against proteinase-3 produce a cytoplasmic staining pattern (cANCA) and antibodies against myeloperoxidase produce perinuclear staining pattern (pANCA). Combined testing by ELISA and indirect immunofluorescence is recommended as this increases specificity at the cost of a 10% reduction of sensitivity. Sometimes antineutrophil cytoplasmic antibody tests are negative, particularly if disease is limited to the upper respiratory tract. Antibody titres usually fall and may disappear completely when the disease is in remission.

Treatment

Treatment of Wegener's granulomatosis and microscopic polyangiitis comprises induction of remission and then maintenance of remission. Multicentre trials are in progress to assess the place of pulse cyclophosphamide, plasma exchange, and methylprednisolone in treatment and to assess the optimum duration of maintenance therapy. Methotrexate is sometimes used instead of cyclophosphamide for patients with no renal disease. Relapses occur in 40-50% of patients during the first five years, so lifelong monitoring for recurring disease activity is essential. The five year survival rate is over 80%.

Churg-Strauss syndrome

Churg-Strauss syndrome is associated with an atopic tendency, usually asthma. It may affect coronary, pulmonary, cerebral, and splanchnic circulations. Rashes with purpura, urticaria, and subcutaneous nodules are common. Glomerulonephritis may develop, but renal failure is uncommon.

Diagnosis depends on presence of typical clinical features, biopsy of skin, lung, and kidney, and blood eosinophilia. About 25% of patients are positive for cANCA, 50% for pANCA, and 25% have no antineutrophil cytoplasmic antibodies.

Many patients respond to high dose corticosteroids alone, although cyclophosphamide may be required for patients with

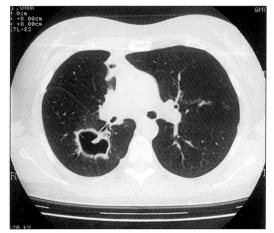
Cavitating granulomatous lesion in right lung of patient with Wegener's granulomatosis

---

Specificity and sensitivity of ANCA serology testing for Wegener's granulomatosis and microscopic polyangiitis (adapted from Hagen et al, *Kidney Int* 1998;53:743-53)

	Specificity/ sensitivity (%)
Specificity of assays (related to disease controls)	
Indirect immunofluorescence:	
cANCA	95
pANCA	81
ELISAs:	
PR3-ANCA	87
MPO-ANCA	91
Combined indirect immunofluorescence and ELISA:	
cANCA/PR3-ANCA positive	99
pANCA/MPO-ANCA positive	99
Sensitivity of combined testing	
Wegener's granulomatosis	73
Microscopic polyangiitis	67

Treatment of small vessel vasculitis

Induction therapy (to 3 months after remission, usually 6 months from diagnosis)
- Cyclophosphamide, 2.0 mg/kg/day (maximum 200 mg/day). Age > 60 years, reduce dose by 25%, > 75 years by 50%
- Prednisolone, 1 mg/kg/day (maximum 80 mg/day) reduced weekly to 25mg/day by 8 weeks and then more slowly to 10 mg/day by 6 months

In severe, life threatening disease (eg, pulmonary haemorrhage, severe crescentic glomerulonephritis with creatinine > 500 µmol/l), consider plasma exchange, 7-10 treatments over 14 days, or three pulses of methylprednisolone, 15 mg/kg/day for 3 days

Maintenance therapy (to 18-24 months, longer if clinically indicated)
- Azathioprine, 2.0 mg/kg/day (maximum 200 mg/day). Age > 60 years, reduce dose by 25%, > 75 years by 50%
- Prednisolone, 5-10 mg/day

Relapse therapy
- Major relapse: return to induction therapy
- Minor relapse: increase dose of corticosteroids

Stop cyclophosphamide or azathioprine if white blood count 4x10⁹/l; restart with a dose reduced by at least 25 mg when white blood count > 4x10⁹/l on two consecutive tests

Consider gastric and bone protection, and fungal and *Pneumocystis carinii* prophylaxis

more severe disease. Asthma requires conventional treatment but the recently introduced leukotriene receptor antagonist drugs have been causally linked with the Churg-Strauss syndrome and should be avoided in these patients.

Small vessel vasculitis without antineutrophil cytoplasmic antibodies

Henoch-Schönlein purpura

Henoch-Schönlein purpura is most common in children but can occur at any age. Typical clinical features are purpura over the lower limbs and buttocks, haematuria, abdominal pain, bloody diarrhoea, and arthralgia. The pathological hallmarks are deposition of immunoglobulin A at the dermoepidermal junction and within the glomerular mesangium, with a mesangial hypercellular glomerulonephritis. Some patients develop a glomerular lesion resembling that seen in small vessel vasculitis. Renal disease may occur without the rash or other typical features.

The disease is usually self limiting and only supportive treatment is required. Corticosteroids and immunosuppression may be needed for vasculitic glomerulonephritis or serious gut haemorrhage and ischaemia.

Cryoglobulinaemic vasculitis ("mixed, essential")

Cryoglobuins are immunoglobulins that precipitate in the cold. The mixed cryoglobulin consists of a monoclonal immunoglobulin M rheumatoid factor complexed to polyclonal immunoglobulin G. Vasculitis develops when cryoglobulins deposit in blood vessels. Mixed essential cryoglobulinaemia is due to hepatitis C virus infection in over 80% of cases. Other causes of cryoglobulinaemia include dysproteinaemias, autoimmune diseases, and chronic infections. Serum complement C4 and C3 concentrations are reduced. Clinical features include palpable purpura, arthralgia, distal necroses, peripheral neuropathy, abdominal pain, and glomerulonephritis. Renal biopsy specimens typically have the appearance of subendothelial membranoproliferative glomerulonephritis with intraglomerular deposits.

In cryoglobulinaemia associated with hepatitis C, treatment is directed at the viral infection. Interferon alfa over six months is beneficial, but many patients relapse when treatment is stopped. Prednisolone with or without immunosuppressants has been used successfully in acute severe disease. The role of plasma exchange remains unsubstantiated.

Isolated cutaneous leukocytoclastic vasculitis

This is often associated with a drug hypersensitivity response and improves when the drug is stopped. Occasional patients may require corticosteroids for severe disease.

Antiglomerular basement membrane antibody mediated disease (Goodpasture's disease)

No Chapel Hill definition exists for this rare disease, which has considerable overlaps with antineutrophil cytoplasmic antibody associated vasculitis. The hallmarks are a rapidly progressive global and diffuse glomerulonephritis, as seen in small vessel vasculitides, or presence of pulmonary haemorrhage, or both. Diagnosis depends on finding antibodies to glomerular basement membrane in the serum and linear staining for immunoglobulin G along the glomerular basement membrane. The antibodies have been implicated in disease pathogenesis. About 15-30% of patients have detectable antineutrophil cytoplasmic antibodies. Treatment is as for small vessel vasculitis with addition of daily plasma exchange until antiglomerular basement membrane antibodies are no longer detectable.

Definitions of non-ANCA associated small vessel vasculitis

Henoch-Schönlein purpura
- Vasculitis with IgA dominant immune deposits affecting small vessels (capillaries, venules, or arterioles)
- Affects skin, gut, and glomeruli
- Associated with arthralgia or arthritis

Cryoglobulinaemic vasculitis
- Vasculitis with cryoglobulin immune deposits affecting small vessels
- Associated with cryoglobulins in serum
- Skin and glomeruli often affected

Isolated cutaneous leukocytoclastic vasculitis
- Isolated cutaneous leukocytoclastic angiitis without systemic vasculitis or glomerulonephritis
- May evolve into systemic vasculitis

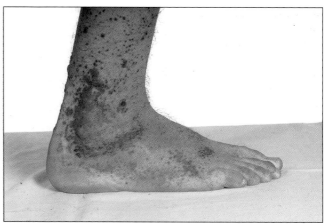

Purpuric rash on lower limb of patient with Henoch-Schönlein purpura

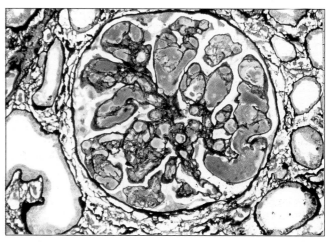

Renal biopsy specimen showing intraglomerular deposit of cryoglobulins

11   Varicose veins

Nick J M London, Roddy Nash

Varicose veins are tortuous, twisted, or lengthened veins. Unless the enlargement is severe, size alone does not indicate abnormality because size can vary depending on ambient temperature and, in women, hormonal factors. In addition, normal superficial veins in a thin person may appear large, whereas varicose veins in an obese person may be hidden. Varicose veins can be classified as trunk, reticular, or telangiectasia. Telangiectasia are also referred to as spider veins, star bursts, thread veins, or matted veins. Most varicose veins are primary; only the minority are secondary to conditions such as deep vein thrombosis and occlusion, pelvic tumours, or arteriovenous fistulae.

Incidence and prevalence

A study of people aged 35 to 70 years in London in 1992 concluded that the prevalence of varicose veins in men and women was 17% and 31% respectively. Although varicose veins have traditionally been considered commoner in women, a recent study from Edinburgh of people aged 18 to 64 years found that the prevalence of trunk varices was 40% in men and 32% in women. Over 80% of the total population had reticular varicosities or telangiectasia. There are few studies on the incidence of varicose veins; however, the Framingham study found that the two year incidence of varicose veins was 39.4/1000 for men and 51.9/1000 for women.

Pathophysiology and risk factors

The theory that varicose veins result from failure of valves in the superficial veins leading to venous reflux and vein dilatation has been superseded by the hypothesis that valve incompetence follows rather than precedes a change in the vein wall. Thus, the vein wall is inherently weak in varicose veins, which leads to dilatation and separation of valve cusps so that they become incompetent. This theory is strongly supported by the observation that the dilatation of varicose veins is initially distal to the valve; if the primary abnormality was descending valve incompetence, the initial dilatation should be proximal to the valve.

Risk factors for varicose veins include increasing age and parity and occupations that require a lot of standing. There is no evidence that social class, smoking, or genetic makeup influence the prevalence of varicose veins. Obesity is associated with the development of varicose veins in women but not in men.

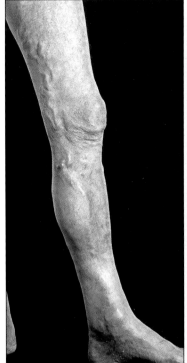
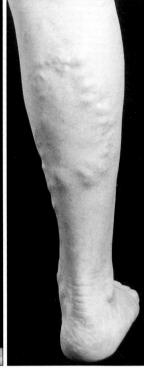

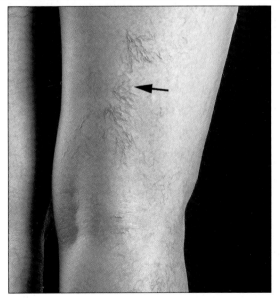

Trunk varices are varicosities in the line of the long (top, left) or short (top, right) saphenous vein or their major branches. Reticular veins (arrow, bottom) are dilated tortuous subcutaneous veins not belonging to the main branches of the long or short saphenous vein, and telangiectasia (bottom) are intradermal venules <1 mm

Symptoms

The Edinburgh vein study recently compared the prevalence of symptoms in men and women with and without varicose veins. In men, the only symptom that was significantly associated with trunk varices was itching, whereas in women, heaviness or tension, aching, and itching were significantly associated with trunk varices. No association was found between reticular varices and lower limb symptoms in either men or women.

Symptoms associated with varicose veins

- Heaviness
- Tension
- Aching
- Itching

Complications of varicose veins

Some complications of varicose veins, such as haemorrhage and thrombophlebitis, result from the varicose veins themselves, whereas others, such as oedema, skin pigmentation, varicose eczema, atrophie blanche, lipodermatosclerosis, and venous ulceration result from venous hypertension. The size of varicose veins does not seem related to the degree of venous hypertension. Indeed, 40% of limbs with ulceration due to superficial venous incompetence do not have visible varicose veins. Venous ulceration is discussed in a subsequent article.

Recurrent varicose veins

In the United Kingdom, about 20% of varicose vein surgery is for recurrence, and the estimated annual cost of such surgery is £11m. Recurrent varicose veins can result from inadequate or defective primary surgery or the development of new sites of reflux. Improved patient assessment and more rigorous primary surgery should reduce the socioeconomic impact of recurrent varicose veins.

Clinical management

History
It is important to determine precisely why the patient has sought treatment. One third of patients presenting with varicose veins have symptoms unrelated to their varicose veins or are worried about deterioration or complications. Such patients simply need reassurance. It is important to determine whether the patient has had deep vein thrombosis or thrombophlebitis and any family history of deep vein thrombosis. History of these conditions increases the risk of deep vein thrombosis after varicose vein surgery and may lead to a decision not to operate. Patients with a history of deep vein thrombosis or thrombophlebitis who have surgery should receive perioperative subcutaneous heparin prophylaxis. It is important to note whether women are taking the contraceptive pill or hormone replacement therapy. Any history of skin changes is also important because affected patients are at high risk of developing ulceration.

Examination and investigation
Examination of the patient should include an abdominal examination to exclude some of the secondary causes of varicose veins. With the patient standing, note the distribution of the varicose veins, in particular whether they are long or short saphenous, or both. Secondary skin changes should be noted. Most vascular surgeons would then investigate the patient in the clinic using handheld Doppler or colour duplex scanning. Although ideally all patients presenting with varicose veins would have colour duplex scanning, the NHS does not have the resources to allow this. Patients with recurrent varicose veins should be scanned to determine the precise site of recurrence. Patients with varicose veins in limbs with a history of deep vein thrombosis or thrombophlebitis should be scanned to make sure that the superficial veins are not acting as collaterals in the presence of deep vein obstruction. Scanning is also essential for patients with venohypertensive skin changes. If the deep veins are competent in the presence of refluxing superficial veins, superficial venous surgery is potentially curative.

Treatment
As discussed above, about a third of patients presenting with varicose veins will require only reassurance or explanation that

Complications of varicose veins
- Haemorrhage
- Thrombophlebitis
- Oedema
- Skin pigmentation
- Atrophie blanche
- Varicose eczema
- Lipodermatosclerosis
- Venous ulceration

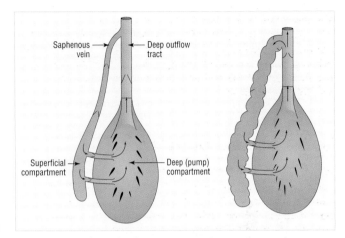

Mechanisms of failure of calf muscle pump and venous hypertenion. Superficial veins do not normally allow reflux of blood (left). However, if superficial veins are incompetent (right), some of the blood ejected by the calf muscle pump during systole refluxes back down the superficial veins into the calf muscle pump during diastole. This retrograde circuit can overload the calf muscle pump, leading to dilatation and failure. The subsequent rise in end diastolic volume leads to venous hypertension. Adapted from Browse et al

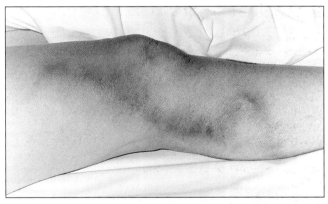

Thrombophlebitis presents as severe pain, erythema, pigmentation over, and hardening of the vein. Thrombophlebitis in varicose veins results from stasis, whereas thrombophlebitis occurring in normal veins should alert clinicians to the possibility of an underlying malignancy or thrombophilia. Recurrent thrombophlebitis in varicose veins raises the possibility of underlying thrombophilia

Indications for colour duplex scanning of varicose veins
- Recurrent varicose veins
- History of superficial thrombophlebitis
- History of deep venous thrombosis
- Varicose eczema
- Haemosiderin staining
- Lipodermatosclerosis
- Venous ulceration

their symptoms are not related to their varicose veins. Patients whose main symptoms are aching or oedema may benefit from compression hosiery. Indeed, if it is uncertain whether the patient's symptoms are caused by varicose veins, a trial of compression hosiery may help; a response to compression indicates that surgery may be beneficial.

The treatment options for trunk varices are injection sclerotherapy or surgery. The use of injection sclerotherapy for trunk varices has fallen in recent years, partly because of concerns about complications such as skin staining and ulceration and also because up to 65% of patients treated by sclerotherapy develop recurrent varicose veins within five years. Currently, sclerotherapy is most commonly used to treat residual varicosities after surgery. Surgery is generally directed at the underlying abnormality, in the form of saphenofemoral or saphenopopliteal disconnection, and in the case of long saphenous varices, stripping of the long saphenous vein with multiple avulsions.

Many patients can be treated as day cases, most can return to driving after one week, and the time off work varies between one and three weeks depending on the patient's occupation. The risk of serious complication (deep venous thrombosis, pulmonary embolism, or arterial or nerve injury) is less than 1%, but roughly 17% of patients will suffer minor complications, most commonly temporary saphenous or sural nerve neuralgia. All patients should be warned of this possibility. After surgery, 20-30% of patients develop recurrent varicose veins within 10 years.

Reticular varices are not connected to major trunk varices and are treated by sclerotherapy or avulsion through small stab incisions. Patients who present with capillary telangiectasia should have colour duplex scanning because roughly 25% will have clinically unapparent long or short saphenous incompetence. The telangiectasia are treated by microinjections, laser, or high intensity light. The last two methods are being increasingly used.

Management of complications

Thrombophlebitis
There is no indication for antibiotics in patients with thrombophlebitis. Patients should be referred to a vascular specialist and surgery considered because thrombophlebitis tends to recur if the underlying venous abnormality is not corrected. Colour duplex studies have shown that up to a quarter of patients with superficial thrombophlebitis have underlying deep venous thrombosis, and it has therefore been suggested that all patients with thombophlebitis should have duplex scanning to exclude deep vein thrombosis. However, a more realistic suggestion is that patients with phlebitis extending up the long saphenous vein towards the saphenofemoral junction should have urgent duplex scanning. If the thrombus extends into the femoral vein, urgent saphenofemoral ligation should be considered.

Bleeding varicose veins
Bleeding varicose veins can be stemmed by raising the foot above the level of the heart and applying compression. The patients should then be seen by a vascular surgeon with a view to correcting the underlying abnormality. If the deep veins are incompetent, the patient should wear compression hosiery.

Varicose eczema, lipodermatosclerosis, and venous ulceration
Patients with varicose eczema or lipodermatosclerosis require colour duplex scanning to define the underlying venous

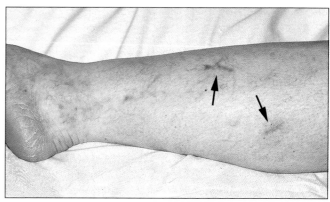

One of the complications of injection sclerotherapy is brown skin pigmentation (arrows)

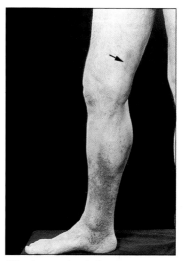

Skin pigmentation is due to haemosiderin deposition. This patient also has thrombophlebitis of the long saphenous vein with overlying pigmentation (arrow)

Management of thrombophlebitis
- Crepe bandaging to compress vein and minimise propogation of thrombus
- Analgesia (preferably non-steroidal anti-inflammatory drug)
- Low dose aspirin

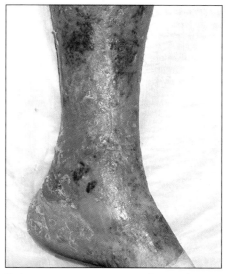

Varicose eczema occurs over prominent varicose veins and in the lower third of the leg. It may be dry, scaly, and vesicular or weeping and ulcerated

abnormality. Generally, if the only abnormality is superficial venous incompetence this should be surgically corrected. If, however, the deep veins are incompetent, then superficial surgery will not help and the patient should be treated with a topical steroid and wear compression hosiery.

Areas of controversy

Whose varicose veins should be treated?

In the absence of clear national guidelines the decision about who should receive varicose vein surgery under the NHS is being made at a local level. In general terms patients with only cosmetic problems are not treated whereas patients with skin changes (eczema, lipodermatosclerosis, and ulceration) are treated. The most controversial group is patients with symptomatic trunk varices and no skin changes. Unfortunately, there is no way of predicting which limbs with varicose veins will subsequently develop venous ulceration, and it is clearly not sensible to operate on the 30% of the population with varicose veins in order to prevent 1% developing an ulcer.

Varicose veins, deep vein thrombosis, contraceptive pill, and hormone replacement therapy

Although varicose veins increase the risk of deep vein thrombosis after major abdominal or orthopaedic surgery, there is no evidence that primary varicose veins are a risk factor for spontaneous deep vein thrombosis. Similarly, there is no evidence that women with varicose veins who take the contraceptive pill or hormone replacement therapy are at increased risk of deep vein thrombosis compared with women without varicose veins. Evidence exists, however, that women with varicose veins who take the pill are more likely to develop thrombophlebitis; a history of thrombophlebitis is therefore a contraindication to the pill and a reason for stopping the pill in current takers. Although not evidence based, the same considerations should probably apply to hormone replacement therapy.

Varicose vein surgery, contraceptive pill, and hormone replacement therapy

Although there is no evidence that varicose vein surgery is high risk for deep vein thrombosis, women taking the combined contraceptive pill or hormone replacement therapy are at increased risk of deep vein thrombosis after varicose vein surgery. Women taking the combined contraceptive pill should either stop the pill four weeks before surgery and restart two weeks later or receive subcutaneous heparin prophylaxis. If the pill is stopped advice must be given about alternative contraception. Women taking hormone replacement therapy should continue taking it and receive heparin thromboprophylaxis.

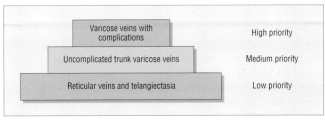

Demand management. High priority cases should be refered for vascular assessment. Many regions are not offering NHS treatment for medium and low priority cases on the basis that resources are needed more for other conditions

Further reading

- Franks PJ, Wright DD, Moffatt CJ, Stirling J, Fletcher AE, Bulpitt CJ, et al. Prevalence of venous disease: a community study in West London. *Eur J Surg* 1992:158:143-7.
- Brand FN, Dannenberg AL, Abbott RD, Kannell WB. The epidemiology of varicose veins: the Framingham study. *Am J Prev Med* 1988;4:96-101.
- Bradbury A, Evans C, Allan P, Lee A, Ruckley CV, Fowkes FGR. What are the symptoms of varicose veins? Edinburgh vein study cross sectional population survey. *BMJ* 1999;318:353-6.
- Campbell B. Thrombosis, phlebitis, and varicose vein surgery. *BMJ* 1996;312:198-9.
- Royal College of General Practitioners' oral contraception study: oral contraceptives, venous thrombosis, and varicose veins. *J R Coll Gen Pract* 1978;28:393-9.
- Drugs in the peri-operative period: 3—Hormonal contraceptives and hormone replacement therapy. *Drug Ther Bull* 1999;37:78-80.
- Tibbs DJ. *Varicose veins and related disorders.* Oxford: Butterworth-Heinemann, 1992.
- Tibbs DJ, Sabiston DC, Davies MG, Mortimer PS, Scurr JH. *Varicose veins, venous disorders, and lymphatic problems in the lower limbs.* Oxford: Oxford University Press, 1997.
- Ruckley CV, Fowkes FGR, Bradbury AW. *Venous disease.* London: Springer-Verlag, 1998.
- Browse NI, Burnand KG, Irvine AT, Wilson NM. *Diseases of the veins.* London: Arnold, 1999.

12 Swollen lower limb–1: General assessment and deep vein thrombosis

W Peter Gorman, Karl R Davis, Richard Donnelly

The most common cause of leg swelling is oedema, but expansion of all or part of a limb may be due to an increase in any tissue component (muscle, fat, blood, etc). A correct diagnosis requires consideration of whether the swelling is acute or chronic, symmetrical or asymmetrical, localised or generalised, and congenital or acquired. Chronic swelling, particularly if asymmetrical, is usually a sign of chronic oedema arising from venous or lymphatic disease, whereas symmetrical lower limb swelling suggests a systemic or more central cause of oedema, such as heart failure or nephrotic syndrome. Oedema develops when the rate of capillary filtration (lymph formation) exceeds lymphatic drainage, either because of increased capillary filtration, inadequate lymphatic flow, or both. Extracellular fluid volume is controlled prinicpally by the lymphatic system, which normally compensates for increases in capillary filtration. Most oedemas arise because filtration overwhelms the lymph drainage system. Increased capillary filtration may occur because of raised venous pressure, hypoalbuminaemia, or increased capillary permeability due to local inflammation. The two main causes of a swollen lower limb are deep vein thrombosis and lymphoedema (a failure of the lymph drainage system). This article concentrates on deep vein thrombosis and next week's article on lymphoedema.

Deep vein thrombosis

Thrombosis usually develops as a result of venous stasis or slow flowing blood around venous valve sinuses; extension of the primary thrombus occurs within or between the deep and superficial veins of the leg and the propagating clot causes venous obstruction, damage to valves, and possible thromboembolism. Deep vein thrombosis is often asymptomatic.

Assessment and investigation

Various clinical features suggest deep vein thrombosis, but the findings of physical examination alone are notoriously unreliable. Deep vein thrombosis is confirmed in only one out of every three cases suspected clinically. Confirmation of a suspected deep vein thrombosis requires use of one or more investigations, and the confirmation rate rises with the number of clinical risk factors. Identification of an underlying cause, if any, will guide both the treatment and the approach to secondary prevention.

Clinical features of acute deep vein thrombosis

- Calf pain or tenderness, or both
- Swelling with pitting oedema
- Swelling below knee in distal deep vein thrombosis and up to groin in proximal deep vein thrombosis
- Increased skin temperature
- Superficial venous dilatation
- Cyanosis can occur with severe obstruction

The standard investigation is contrast venography, but this invasive procedure is painful, often technically difficult and time consuming, and occasionally complicated by thrombosis and

---

Causes of swelling of lower limb

Acute
- Deep vein thrombosis
- Cellulitis
- Superficial thrombophlebitis
- Joint effusion or haemarthrosis
- Haematoma
- Baker's cyst
- Torn gastrocnemius muscle
- Arthritis
- Fracture
- Acute arterial ischaemia
- Dermatitis

Chronic

Congenital vascular abnormalities
- Haemangioma
- Klippel-Trenaunay syndrome

Venous disease
- Post-thrombotic syndrome
- Lipodermatosclerosis
- Chronic venous insufficiency
- Venous obstruction

Lymphoedema
- Cancer treatment
- Infection
- Tumour
- Trauma
- Pretibial myxoedema

Other
- Heart failure
- Reflex sympathetic dystrophy
- Idiopathic oedema of women
- Hypoproteinaemia, such as cirrhosis, nephrotic syndrome
- Armchair legs
- Lipoedema

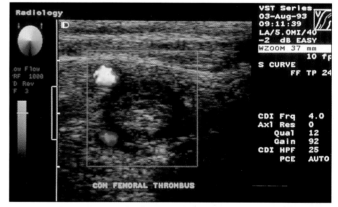

Colour duplex scan of deep vein thrombosis in common femoral vein adjacent to artery

---

Risk factors for deep vein thrombosis

- Age >40 years
- Underlying malignancy
- Obesity
- Presence of varicose veins
- Personal or family history of deep vein thrombosis or pulmonary embolism
- Any surgical procedure lasting more than 30 minutes—especially orthopaedic, neurosurgical, urological, and gynaecological surgery
- Paralysis or immobility—for example, recent stroke
- Combined contraceptive pill
- Hormone replacement therapy
- Pregnancy and puerperium
- Serious illness—for example, heart failure, myocardial infarction, sepsis, inflammatory bowel disease
- Presence of hypercoagulable disorders

extravasation of contrast. Recent developments in non-invasive testing mean that venography is now unnecessary in most cases, particularly in suspected first proximal vein thrombosis.

The accuracy of non-invasive techniques varies with the clinical circumstances. For example, compression ultrasonography and impedance plethysmography are accurate for detecting symptomatic proximal (ileofemoral) deep vein thrombosis, but both techniques are less satisfactory in asymptomatic patients and for detecting distal (calf vein) thrombosis. Compression ultrasonography has become the preferred first line investigation (see *BMJ* 2000;320:698-701).

Imaging techniques are generally much less satisfactory in patients with suspected recurrent deep vein thrombosis, when confirmation of the diagnosis requires evidence of new thrombus formation—for example, the appearance of a new non-compressible venous segment on ultrasonography or a new intraluminal filling defect on venography.

Measurement of circulating D-dimer concentrations (a byproduct of fibrin production) is a useful adjunct to ultrasonography, with 98% sensitivity for deep vein thrombosis and a high negative predictive value. The sensitivity of the test is lower for smaller calf vein thrombi. However D-dimer concentrations rise as a non-specific response to concomitant illness, not just thrombosis, so D-dimer testing can be misleading in patients admitted to hospital for other reasons.

A combination of diagnostic approaches—for example, compression ultrasonography coupled with clinical pretest probability scoring or D-dimer measurements, or both, gives better diagnostic accuracy than any single investigation. Lensing et al have recently shown that the combination of compression ultrasonography and D-dimer measurement is an efficient diagnostic approach, with a rate of subsequent thromboembolism less than 1% in patients with false negative results who were not treated with heparin. A robust investigational algorithm has been devised that does not include routine use of venography.

Complications

The main complications of deep vein thrombosis are pulmonary embolism, post-thrombotic syndrome, and recurrence of thrombosis. Proximal thrombi are a major source of morbidity and mortality. Distal thrombi are generally smaller and more difficult to detect non-invasively, and their prognosis and clinical importance are less clear. However, a fifth of untreated newly developing calf vein thrombi extend proximally, and a quarter are associated with long term symptoms of post-thrombotic syndrome; it is therefore appropriate to treat proved significant calf vein thrombosis.

Post-thrombotic syndrome develops as a result of high venous pressure due to thrombotic damage to valves. It complicates 50-75% of deep vein thromboses, and there is a strong association with ipsilateral recurrence. Clinical features include pain, swelling, dermatitis, and ulceration. Proximal deep vein thrombosis is associated with a higher frequency and greater severity of post-thrombotic syndrome, but the risk is halved by use of graded compression stockings after deep vein thrombosis.

Prevention

Patients at significantly increased risk of deep vein thrombosis—for example, those having major pelvic or abdominal surgery for cancer or those with a history of pulmonary embolism or deep vein thrombosis who have

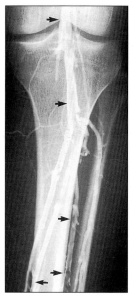

Venogram showing thrombus in lower leg

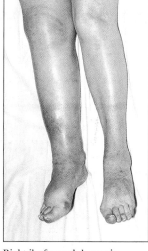

Right ileofemoral deep vein thrombosis

Clinical model to determine pretest probability of deep vein thombosis (3 points=high risk, 1 or 2=moderate, 0=low)

	Score
Active cancer (treatment ongoing, or within 6 months, or palliative)	1
Paralysis, paresis or recent plaster immobilisation of the legs	1
Recent immobilisation > 3days or major surgery within 12 weeks requiring general or regional anaesthesia	1
Localised tenderness along the distribution of the deep venous system	1
Entire leg swollen	1
Calf swelling >3 cm than asymptomatic side (measured 10 cm below tibial tuberosity)	1
Pitting oedema confined to the symptomatic leg	1
Collateral superficial veins (non-varicose)	1
Alternative diagnosis equally or more likely than deep vein thrombosis	− 2

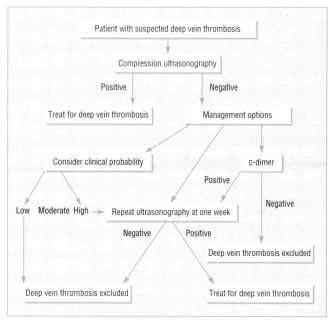

Algorithm for investigation of deep vein thrombosis

Absolute risks of venous thrombotic complications in procedures or conditions of low, moderate, and high risk

Risk level	Risk (%)			Examples
	Deep vein thrombosis	Proximal deep vein thrombosis	Fatal pulmonary embolism	
Low	< 10	< 1	0.01	Minor surgery, trauma, or medical illness Major surgery at age < 40 with no other risk factors
Moderate	10-40	1-10	0.1-1	Major surgery with another risk factor Major trauma, medical illness, or burns Emergency caesarean section in labour Minor surgery with previous deep vein thrombosis, pulmonary embolism, or thrombophilia Lower limb paralysis
High	40-80	10-30	1-10	Major pelvic or abdominal surgery for cancer Major surgery, trauma, or illness with previous pulmonary embolish, deep vein thrombosis, or thrombophilia

serious trauma or illness or are having major surgery—should be given prophylaxis. Early mobilisation and graduated compression stockings are effective, and antiplatelet drugs such as aspirin provide additional protection.

Pneumatic compression devices have been proved effective when used perioperatively and in some groups of medical patients. Low dose unfractionated heparin (5000 units two hours before surgery and 8-12 hourly postoperatively) given by subcutaneous injection reduces the rate of postoperative thromboembolism in general surgical patients by 65%, with little increase in the risk of serious bleeding. Low molecular weight heparins are effective and have some advantages over unfractionated heparin, particularly in high risk patients such as those having hip replacement.

Treatment

Treatment is aimed at reducing symptoms and preventing complications. Elevation of the leg with some flexion at the knee helps reduce swelling, early mobilisation is beneficial, and use of graded compression stockings achieves a 60% reduction in post-thrombotic syndrome.

It is important to establish effective anticoagulation rapidly. Patients are usually given an intial intravenous heparin bolus of 5000 units followed by unfractionated or low molecular weight heparin for at least five days. With unfractionated heparin an intravenous constant infusion and subcutaneaous injection twice daily are equally effective. A heparin algorithm should be used to adjust the dose. The activated partial thromboplastin time should be checked six hourly until the target is reached and then daily to maintain the international normalised ratio at 1.5-2.5. The platelet count should be checked at the start of treatment and on day 5 to exclude thrombocytopenia. Warfarin should be started on day 1, with the dose determined by a warfarin algorithm. The target ratio is 2-3, and heparin can be stopped when the target ratio is maintained for more than 24 hours.

Patients with deep vein thrombosis who do not need to be in hospital (around 35%) can be treated with subcutaneous low molecular weight heparin in the community. This can be administered subcutaneously once or twice daily. Low molecular weight heparin has the advantages of a slightly lower rate of haemorrhage and thrombocytopenia and more reliable absorption after injection, and anticoagulation monitoring is not required routinely. Warfarin should be started on day 1, and the duration of treatment guided by the risk profile.

Other approaches
Inferior vena cava filters reduce the rate of pulmonary embolism but have no effect on the other complications of deep

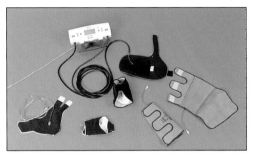
Pneumatic compression devices

Duration of anticoagulation in patients with deep vein thrombosis

- Transient cause and no other risk factors: 3 months
- Idiopathic: 3-6 months
- Ongoing risk—for example, malignancy: 6-12 months
- Recurrent pulmonary embolism or deep vein thrombosis: 6-12 months
- Patients with high risk of recurrent thrombosis exceeding risk of anticoagulation: indefinite duration (subject to review)

Indications for insertion of an inferior vena cava filter

- Pulmonary embolism with contraindication to anticoagulation
- Recurrent pulmonary embolism despite adequate anticoagulation
Controversial indications:
- Deep vein thrombosis with contraindication to anticoagulation
- Deep vein thrombosis in patients with pre-existing pulmonary hypertension
- Free floating thrombus in proximal vein
- Failure of existing filter device
- Post pulmonary embolectomy

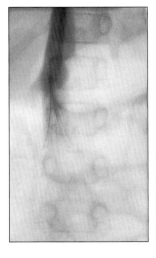
Vena cavagram showing umbrella delivery device inserted into the inferior vena cava through the jugular vein. The filter has been released just below the renal veins. Inferior vena cava filters help prevent pulmonary embolism but not other complications of deep vein thrombosis, including recurrent thrombosis

vein thrombosis. Thrombolysis should be considered in patients with major proximal vein thrombosis and threatened venous infarction. Surgical embolectomy is restricted to life threatening proximal thrombosis where all else has failed.

Pregnancy

Anticoagulating doses of heparin are given for deep vein thrombosis in pregnancy. It is essential to confirm the presence of a thrombus objectively. This is usually done by compression ultrasonography (serially if necessary).

Unfractionated heparin or low molecular weight heparin (which has a better risk profile but is not licensed in United Kingdom for this indication) should then be continued throughout the pregnancy and stopped temporarily before delivery. Anticoagulation should be restarted in the puerperium and continued for six weeks to three months. Warfarin is usually contraindicated during pregnancy because it is teratogenic and increases risk of maternal and fetal haemorrhage perinatally. It can be restarted 48 hours after delivery.

Further reading and useful references

- Levick JR. *An introduction to cardiovascular physiology.* 2nd ed. Oxford: Butterworth-Heinemann, 1995.
- Lensing WA, Prandoni P, Prins MH, Buller HR. Deep vein thrombosis. *Lancet* 1999;353:479-85.
- Second Thromboembolic Risk Factors (THRiFT II) Consensus Group. Risk of and prophylaxis for venous thromboembolism in hospital patients. *Phlebology* 1998;13:87-97.
- Kearon C, Julian JA, Math M, Newman TE, Ginsberg JS. Non-invasive diagnosis of deep venous thrombosis. *Ann Intern Med* 1998;128:663-77.
- Anderson DR, Wells PS. Improvements in the diagnostic approach for patients with suspected deep vein thrombosis or pulmonary embolism. *Thromb Haemost* 1999;82:878-86.
- Prins MH, Hutten BA, Koopman MMW, Buller HR. Long-term treatment of venous thromboembolic disease. *Thromb Haemost* 1999;82:892-8.

Deep vein thrombosis in pregnancy and puerperium and in women taking contraceptive pill or hormone replacement therapy

- Normal pregnancy is a hypercoagulable state
- Deep vein thrombosis occurs antepartum in 0.6/1000 women aged < 35 years and 1.2/1000 women >35 and postpartum in 0.3/1000 and 0.7/1000 respectively
- Age, operative delivery, personal or family history, and thrombophilia are particular risks
- Heparin does not cross the placenta and is not secreted in breast milk
- Prolonged heparin therapy raises concerns about osteoporosis, heparin-induced thrombocytopenia, and allergy
- The combined contraceptive pill increases the relative risk of deep vein thrombosis by 3-4 times
- Hormone replacement therapy also increases the relative risk of deep vein thrombosis by 3-4 times but is associated with a 10 fold higher absolute risk because of the older age group

13 Swollen lower limb–2: Lymphoedema

Peter S Mortimer

Lymph conducting pathways may become reduced in number, obliterated, obstructed, or dysfunctional (because of failure of contractility or valve incompetence). A lack of sensitive methods for investigation makes it difficult to distinguish between these mechanisms. A defect in the lymph conducting pathways leads to primary lymphoedema; in practice this means no identifiable outside cause can be found. Secondary lymphoedema is due to factors originating outside the lymphatic system.

Primary lymphoedema

Congenital lymphoedema presenting at or soon after birth is rare. A family history suggests Milroy's disease. Swelling invariably affects both lower limbs, but the upper limbs and face may also swell.

Limb swelling may be the presenting and major manifestation of congenital lymphatic malformations either in a pure form—for example, diffuse lymphangioma—or in combination with a congenital vascular syndrome—for example, Klippel-Trenaunay syndrome (varicose veins, excessive long bone growth, and vascular birthmark).

Most forms of primary lymphoedema present after puberty with foot and ankle swelling. Women are more often affected, and the condition may be familial—for example, Meige's disease. Lymph reflux due to lymphatic vessel hypertrophy or megalymphatics is clinically distinguishable.

Secondary lymphoedema

Lymphoedema manifesting with sudden onset of swelling of one whole leg suggests proximal obstruction. Pelvic causes of venous or lymphatic obstruction such as tumour or thrombosis must be excluded. In the Western world cancer treatment—for example, surgery or radiotherapy) is the commonest cause. Cancer itself rarely presents with lymphoedema except in advanced cases presenting late, such as prostate cancer, where venous obstruction may coexist. Relapsed tumour should always be considered in someone with limb swelling after apparent curative cancer treatment.

Filariasis is probably the most common cause of secondary lymphoedema worldwide and should be considered in any patient with lymphoedema who has travelled or lived in an endemic area.

Clinical diagnosis of lymphoedema

The clinical diagnosis of lymphoedema depends on the history and characteristic skin changes. Although most swelling occurs in the subcutaneous layer, the skin becomes thicker (as demonstrated by the inablity to pinch a fold of skin at the base of the second toe), skin creases become enhanced, and a warty texture (hyperkeratosis) and papillomatosis develop. Such skin changes are termed "elephantiasis."

The differential diagnosis includes venous oedema, "armchair legs," and lipodystrophy or lipoedema, which is often misdiagnosed as lymphoedema.

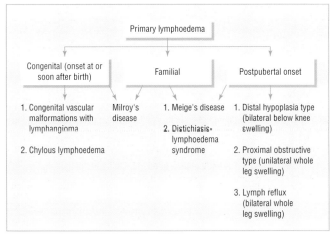

Classification of primary lymphoedema

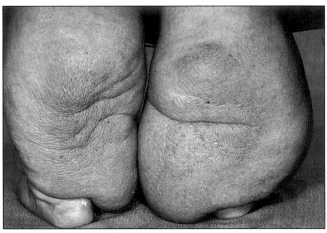

Primary lymphoedema with bilateral below knee swelling due to hypoplasia of peripheral lymphatic vessels

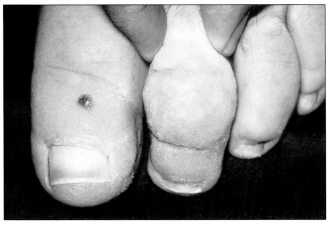

Kaposi-Stemmer sign: inability to pinch a fold of skin at base of second toe because of thickened skin indicates lymphoedema

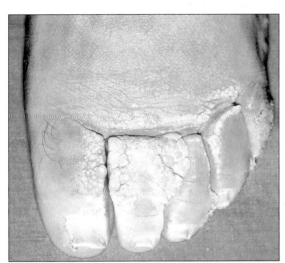

Dilatation of upper dermal lymphatics with consequent fibrosis gives rise to papillomatosis

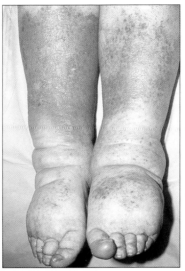

Armchair legs (elephantiasis nostras verrucosis) develop in patients who sit in a chair day and night with their legs dependent. Patients with with cardiac or respiratory disease, stroke, spinal damage, or arthritis are predisoposed to this condition

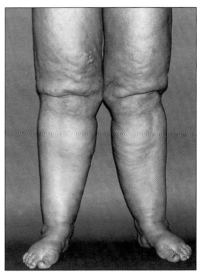

Lipoedema only affects women and causes swelling between hip and ankle with sparing of the foot. The condition is symmetrical. The skin and subcutaneous tissues are soft and often tender with easy bruising

Investigation of lymphoedema

Lymphoscintigraphy (isotope lymphography)
Lymphoscintigraphy is the best investigation for identifying oedema of lymphatic origin. Radiolabelled colloid or protein is injected into the first web space of each foot and monitored using a gamma camera as it moves to the draining lymph nodes. Measurement of tracer uptake within the lymph nodes after a defined interval will distinguish lymphoedema from oedema of non-lymphatic origin. The appearance of tracer outside the main lymph routes, particularly in the skin (dermal backflow), indicates lymph reflux and suggests proximal obstruction. Poor transit of isotope from the injection site suggests hypoplasia of the peripheral lymphatic system.

Direct contrast x ray lymphography (lymphangiography)
After the lymph vessels have been identified with a vital dye, a contrast medium such as Lipiodol is administered directly into a peripheral lymphatic vessel, usually in the dorsum of the foot. In a normal limb the lymphangiogram will show opacification of five to 15 main collecting vessels as they converge on the lowermost inguinal lymph nodes. In patients with lymphatic obstruction the contrast medium will often reflux into the dermal network, so called "dermal backflow."

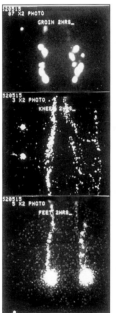

Lymphoscintigraphy. Radiolabelled colloid or protein is injected into the first web space of each foot and followed with a gamma camera as it moves to the draining lymph nodes. Tracer can be seen within the main lymphatic channels and lymph nodes as well as within the infection site. Collateral drainage is seen within the left thigh

Computed tomography and magnetic resonance imaging
Both computed tomography and magnetic resonance imaging detect a characteristic "honeycomb" pattern in the subcutaneous compartment that is not seen with other causes of oedema. In post-thrombotic syndrome the muscle compartment deep to the fascia is enlarged, whereas in lymphoedema it is unchanged. Thickening of the skin is also characteristic of lymphoedema, although it is not diagnostic. Magnetic resonance imaging is more informative than computed tomography because it can detect water.

Management of lymphoedema

Most patients with lymphoedema are just told to live with it, but this is neither necessary nor acceptable.

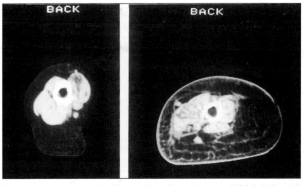

Computed tomogram showing sections through normal thigh (left) and thigh with lymphoedema (right). Note thickened skin and honeycomb pattern

ABC of Arterial and Venous Disease

Physical treatment to reduce swelling
Treatment is aimed at controlling lymph formation and improving lymph drainage through existing lymphatic vessels and collateral routes by applying normal physiological processes which stimulate lymph flow.

Prevention of infection
Prevention of acute inflammatory episodes (cellulitis or lymphangitis) is crucial because they can cause severe constitutional upset and deterioration in swelling. Care of the skin, good hygiene, control of skin diseases such as tinea pedis, and careful antiseptic dressings after minor wounds are all important. Antibiotics must be given promptly when an acute inflammatory episode occurs. In recurrent cellulitis the only effective treatment is prophylactic antibiotics—for example, phenoxymethylpenicillin 500 mg daily, for an indefinite period.

Drug treatment for lymphoedema
Diuretics are of little benefit in lymphoedema because their main action is to limit capillary filtration. Improvement in patients who are taking diuretics suggests that the predominant cause of the oedema is not lymphatic. The benefit of benzopyrones, such as coumarin or flavonoids, remains unproved.

Surgery
Surgery is of value in a few patients in whom the size and weight of a limb inhibit its use and interfere with mobility after physical treatment. Surgery is aimed at either removing excessive tissue (reducing or debulking operations) or bypassing local lymphatic defects.

Further reading
- Ko DS, Lerner R, Klose G, Cosimi AB. Effective treatment of lymphedema of the extremities. *Arch Surg* 1998;133:452-8.
- Mortimer PS. The swollen limb and lymphatic problems. In: Tibbs DJ, Sabiston DC, Davies MG, Mortimer PS, Scurr JH. *Varicose veins, venous disorders and lymphatic problems in the lower limb.* Oxford: Oxford University Press, 1997.
- Levick JR. *An introduction to cardiovascular physiology.* 2nd ed. Oxford: Butterworth-Henemann, 1995.

Physical treatment for lymphoedema

Process	Effect
Exercise	Dynamic muscle contractions encourage both passive (movement of lymph along tissue planes and non-contractile lymph vessels) and active (increased contractility of collecting lymph vessels) drainage
Compression (hosiery)	Opposes capillary filtration. Acts as a counterforce to muscle contractions (so generating greater interstitial pressure changes)
Manual lymphatic drainage	Form of massage that stimulates lymph flow in more proximal, normally draining lymphatics to "siphon" lymph from congested areas (particularly trunk)
Multilayer bandaging	Used as an intensive treatment in combination with exercise to reduce large, misshapen lower limbs and permit subsequent maintenance treatment with hosiery
Pneumatic compression	Softens and reduces limb volume but can forcibly displace fluid into trunk and genitalia. Hosiery must always be worn afterwards
Elevation	Does not stimulate lymph drainage but lowers venous pressure and therefore filtration, allowing lymph drainage to catch up

14 Ulcerated lower limb

Nick J M London, Richard Donnelly

Ulceration of the lower limb affects 1% of the adult population and 3.6% of people older than 65 years. Leg ulcers are debilitating and painful and greatly reduce patients' quality of life. Ulcer healing has been shown to restore quality of life. Lower limb ulceration tends to be recurrent, and the total annual cost of leg ulceration to the NHS has been estimated at £400m.

Aetiology

Venous disease, arterial disease, and neuropathy cause over 90% of lower limb ulcers. It is useful to divide leg ulcers into those occurring in the gaiter area and those occurring in the forefoot because the aetiologies in these two sites are different. At least two aetiological factors can be identified in one third of all lower limb ulcers.

Venous ulcers most commonly occur above the medial or lateral malleoli. Arterial ulcers often affect the toes or shin or occur over pressure points. Neuropathic ulcers tend to occur on the sole of the foot or over pressure points. Apart from necrobiosis lipoidica, diabetes is not a primary cause of ulceration but often leads to ulceration through neuropathy or ischaemia or both. The possibility of malignancy, particularly in ulcers that fail to start healing after adequate treatment, should always be borne in mind. The commonest malignancies are basal cell carcinoma, squamous cell carcinoma, and melanoma.

Patients with reduced mobility or obesity may develop ulceration in the gaiter area because of venous hypertension resulting from inadequate functioning of the calf muscle pump. The commonest causes of vasculitic ulcers are rheumatoid arthritis, systemic lupus, and polyarteritis nodosa. The blood dyscrasias that most commonly lead to leg ulceration are sickle cell disease, thalassaemia, thrombocythaemia, and polycythaemia rubra vera.

Clinical assessment

History
It is important to determine the duration of ulceration and whether it is a first episode or recurrent. Pain is a major problem for patients with leg ulcers unless there is a neuropathic component. Lack of pain therefore suggests a neuropathic aetiology. Systemic diseases that may contribute to the development of the leg ulceration (such as diabetes or rheumatoid arthritis) should be noted, as should a history of trauma, deep venous thrombosis, or varicose vein treatment. Patients should also be asked about their mobility.

Examination
Examination of the leg should include palpation of pulses and a search for the signs of venous hypertension, including varicose veins, haemosiderin pigmentation, varicose eczema, atrophie blanche, and lipodermatosclerosis. The range of hip, knee, and ankle movement should be determined and sensation should be tested—for example, with a monofilament—to exclude a peripheral neuropathy.

In patients with ulcers on the sole of the foot, the sole should be examined for signs of ascending infection, including proximal tenderness and appearance of pus on proximal compression of the sole. Note any surrounding callus typical of

Causes of lower limb ulceration

- Venous disease
- Arterial disease
- Mixed venous-arterial disease
- Neuropathy
- Trauma
- Obesity or immobility
- Vasculitis
- Malignancy
- Underlying osteomyelitis
- Blood dyscrasias
- Lymphoedema
- Necrobiosis lipoidica diabetecorum
- Pyoderma gangrenosum
- Self inflicted

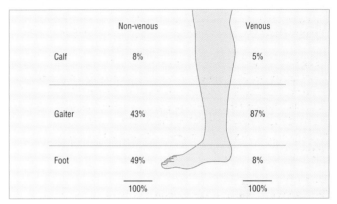

Distribution of non-venous and venous ulcers of lower limb. The majority of venous ulcers are in the gaiter area and the majortiy of non-venous ulcers in foot

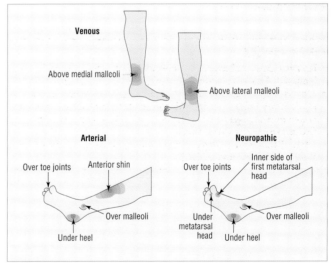

Common sites of venous, arterial, and neuropathic ulceration. Adapted from Tibbs et al

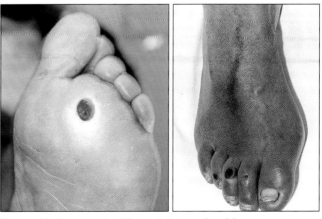

Neuropathic ulcers on sole of foot and dorsum of toe joints

53

neuropathic ulceration and look for tracking to affect the bones of the foot.

Investigation

Patients with foot ulceration should be referred to hospital for investigation because many will have underlying arterial ischaemia that requires prompt intervention. Diabetic patients with signs of infection should have plain radiography of the foot to look for osteomyelitis. Patients with venous ulceration should have their ankle brachial pressure index measured and can be managed either primarily in the community by trained nurses or referred to hospital for further investigation into the underlying venous abnormality.

Management

The management of the more unusual causes of lower leg ulceration is based on treating the underlying disease. However, because venous disease affects up to 30% of the population, it is not uncommon for patients with, for example, rheumatoid arthritis to have lower limb ulceration caused by venous disease. Indeed, in up to half of patients with rheumatoid arthritis and leg ulcers the ulceration is due to venous disease rather than to the rheumatoid arthritis.

Venous ulceration

Debate continues not only about how venous ulcers should be treated but also where they should be treated. It has recently been suggested that patients with leg ulcers should have an initial assessment in a hospital vascular clinic, with patients who are unlikely to benefit from surgery then being cared for in the community. Although this approach has the potential for large cost savings, clinical trials are required to establish cost effectiveness. There is no evidence that any form of drug treatment improves venous ulcer healing, and antibiotics should be used only if the patient has cellulitis.

Community management

Current evidence suggests that the mainstay of the community management of venous ulceration should be graduated compression bandaging. The compression bandaging should be elastic and have multiple layers with a simple, non-adherent dressing underneath. For compression bandaging to be safely applied the ankle brachial pressure index must be at least 0.8. Nurses caring for patients with venous ulcer need to be trained to measure the ankle brachial pressure index and apply compression bandages safely. The bandages should be changed once or twice a week. The healing rate depends on the initial size of the ulcer, but 65-70% of venous ulcers heal within 6 months.

The skin on the lower leg should be kept moist with an emollient such as simple aqueous cream or 50:50 liquid: white paraffin, and surrounding eczema should be treated with a topical steroid. It is important to keep both the primary wound dressing and any medicaments used as "bland" as possible because many patients with venous ulcers develop a contact dermatitis to wound care products.

Hospital treatment

Patients referred to a hospital clinic will have colour duplex scanning to define the underlying venous abnormality. Recent studies have shown that about 60% of patients with venous ulcers have isolated superficial venous incompetence with normal deep veins. Evidence is mounting that patients with long saphenous or short saphenous incompetence in the presence of normal deep veins should have surgery to correct the venous

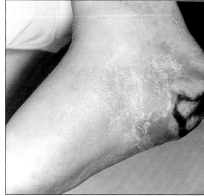
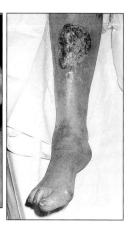
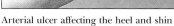

Arterial ulcer affecting the heel and shin

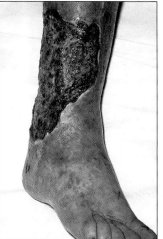
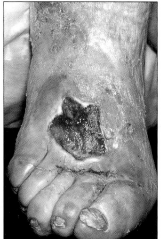

Venous ulcers usually occur above the malleoli (left) but may affect the dorsum of the foot (right)

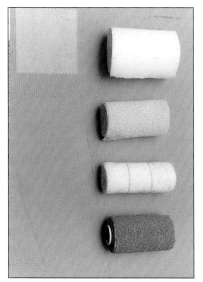
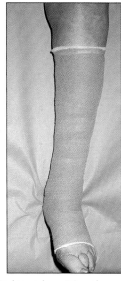

Components of Charing Cross four layer bandaging regimen. The primary wound dressing (left) is a non-adherent dressing, over which are placed (middle; top to bottom in order of use) wool, crêpe, Elset, and Coban bandages. The bandages (right) need replacing once or twice a week

abnormality in the leg and allow ulcer healing. Patients with refluxing deep veins do not benefit from superficial venous surgery and are best managed by compression bandaging in the community.

Prevention of recurrence
The five year recurrence rate of healed venous ulcers can be as high as 40%, and preventing recurrence is therefore very important. The rate of recurrence in patients who have had surgery to correct superficial venous incompetence has not yet been established, but is expected to be low. In patients with healed ulcers who have not had surgery, the mainstay of preventing recurrence is graduated elastic compression hosiery. One study found that ulcers recurred in 19% of patients wearing class 2 compression hosiery compared with 69% of non-compliant patients. However, elderly patients with arthritis of the knee or hip may struggle to apply class 2 compression hosiery, and class 1 hosiery is a sensible compromise. Such patients may find a hosiery applicator useful.

Arterial ulceration
In order for arterial ulcers to heal, the underlying arterial abnormality must be corrected. Patients therefore require colour duplex scanning of their arterial system or diagnostic arteriography to define the underlying arterial abnormality. Angioplasty is the treatment of choice because bypass grafting in patients with ulcers carries an increased risk of wound or graft infection. For patients in whom angioplasty is not possible, some form of bypass operation, preferably using the saphenous vein, should be attempted.

Neuropathic ulceration
The commonest cause of neuropathic ulceration is diabetes, and many diabetic patients with neuropathic ulceration will also have an arterial problem that requires correction. In many hospitals diabetic patients with foot ulcers are managed in specialist foot clinics run by a combination of diabetes physicians, vascular surgeons, specialist nurses, and podiatrists. The principles behind treatment are to optimise blood supply, debride callus and dead tissue, treat active infection, and protect the ulcerated area so that healing can occur. This often requires the use of a protective plaster boot with a window cut out at the site of the ulcer. Once healing has occurred, the patient is fitted with footwear designed to minimise trauma and protect bony prominences.

Key references
- Ruckley CV. Caring for patients with chronic leg ulcer. *BMJ* 1998;316:407-8.
- Scottish Intercollegiate Guidelines Network. The care of patients with chronic leg ulcer. *SIGN 26.* July 1998.
- Fletcher A, Cullum N, Sheldon TA. Systematic review of compression treatment for venous leg ulcers. *BMJ* 1997;315:576-80.
- Scriven JM, Hartshorne T, Bell PRF, Naylor AR, London NJM. Single-visit venous ulcer assessment clinic: the first year. *Br J Surg* 1997;84:334-6.
- Tibbs DJ, Sabiston DC, Davies MG, Mortimer PS, Scurr JH. *Varicose veins, venous disorders, and lymphatic problems in the lower limbs.* Oxford: Oxford University Press, 1997.
- Ruckley CV, Fowkes FGR, Bradbury AW. *Venous disease.* London: Springer-Verlag, 1998.
- Browse Nl, Burnand KG, Irvine AT, Wilson NM. *Diseases of the veins.* London: Arnold, 1999.
- Task Force on Chronic Venous Disorders of the Leg. The management of chronic venous disorders of the leg. *Phlebology* 1999;14(suppl 1).

Classes of compression stocking: most patients can be managed with below knee class 2 stockings

Class	Pressure at ankle (mm Hg)	Uses
1	14-17	Mild varicose veins
2	18-24	Treatment and prevention of venous ulcer recurrence
3	25-35	Treatment of severe venous hypertension and ulcer prevention in large diameter calves

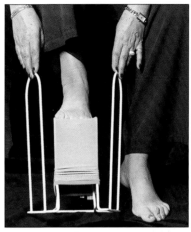
Patients may find an applicator helps with putting on compression hosiery

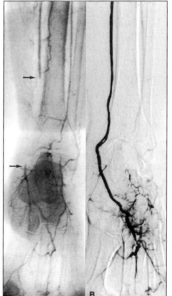
Occlusion (arrows) of distal posterior tibial artery before (left) and after angioplasty (right)

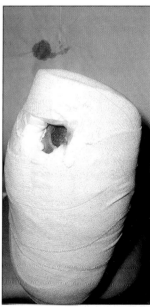
Protective plaster boot with window cut out

Index

Page references in **bold** refer to artwork

Index

Titles in the ABC series from BMJ Books

ABC of AIDS (4th edition)
Edited by Michael W Adler

ABC of Alcohol (3rd edition)
Alex Paton

ABC of Allergies
Edited by Stephen R Durham

ABC of Antenatal Care (3rd edition)
Geoffrey Chamberlain

ABC of Asthma (4th edition)
John Rees and Dipak Kanabar

ABC of Atrial Fibrillation
Edited by Gregory Y H Lip

ABC of Brain Stem Death (2nd edition)
C Pallis and D H Harley

ABC of Breast Diseases
Edited by Michael Dixon

ABC of Child Abuse (3rd edition)
Edited by Roy Meadow

ABC of Clinical Genetics (revised 2nd edition)
Helen Kingston

ABC of Clinical Haematology
Drew Provan and Andrew Henson

ABC of Colorectal Diseases (2nd edition)
Edited by D J Jones

ABC of Dermatology (3rd edition)
Paul K Buxton

ABC of Dermatology (Hot Climates edition)
Paul K Buxton

ABC of Diabetes (4th edition)
Peter Watkins

ABC of Emergency Radiology
Edited by D Nicholson and P Driscoll

ABC of Eyes (3rd edition)
P T Khaw and A R Elkington

ABC of Healthy Travel (5th edition)
Eric Walker, Glyn Williams, Fiona Raeside and Lorna Calvert

ABC of Hypertension (3rd edition)
E O'Brien, D G Beevers and H Marshall

ABC of Intensive Care
Edited by Mervyn Singer and Ian Grant

ABC of Labour Care
G Chamberlain, P Steer and L Zander

ABC of Major Trauma (3rd edition)
Edited by David Skinner and Peter Driscoll

ABC of Medical Computing
Nicholas Lee and Andrew Millman

ABC of Mental Health
Edited by Teifion Davies and T K J Craig

ABC of Monitoring Drug Therapy
J K Aronson, M Hardman and D J M Reynolds

ABC of Nutrition (3rd edition)
A Stewart Truswell

ABC of One to Seven (4th edition)
H B Valman

ABC of Otolaryngology (4th edition)
Harold Ludman

ABC of Palliative Care
Edited by Marie Fallon and Bill O'Neill

ABC of Resuscitation (4th edition)
Edited by M C Colquhoun, A J Handley and T R Evans

ABC of Rheumatology (2nd edition)
Edited by Michael L Snaith

ABC of Sexual Health
Edited by John Tomlinson

ABC of Sexually Transmitted Diseases (4th edition)
Michael W Adler

ABC of Spinal Cord Injury (3rd edition)
David Grundy and Andrew Swain

ABC of Sports Medicine (2nd edition)
Edited by G McLatchie, M Harries, C Williams and J King

ABC of Transfusion (3rd edition)
Edited by Marcela A Contreras

ABC of Urology
Chris Dawson and Hugh Whitfield

ABC of Vascular Diseases
Edited by John Wolfe

ABC of Work Related Disorders
Edited by David Snashall

The First Year of Life (4th edition)
H B Valman

To order, please contact BMJ Bookshop, PO Box 295, London WC1H 9TE, UK
Tel: +44 (0)20 7383 6244   **Fax**: +44 (0)20 7383 6455   **Email**: orders@bmjbookshop.com